30 DAYS PLANT-BASED DIET FOR AGING

The secrets of aging gracefully with a vegan lifestyle

Dr Evelyn James O.K

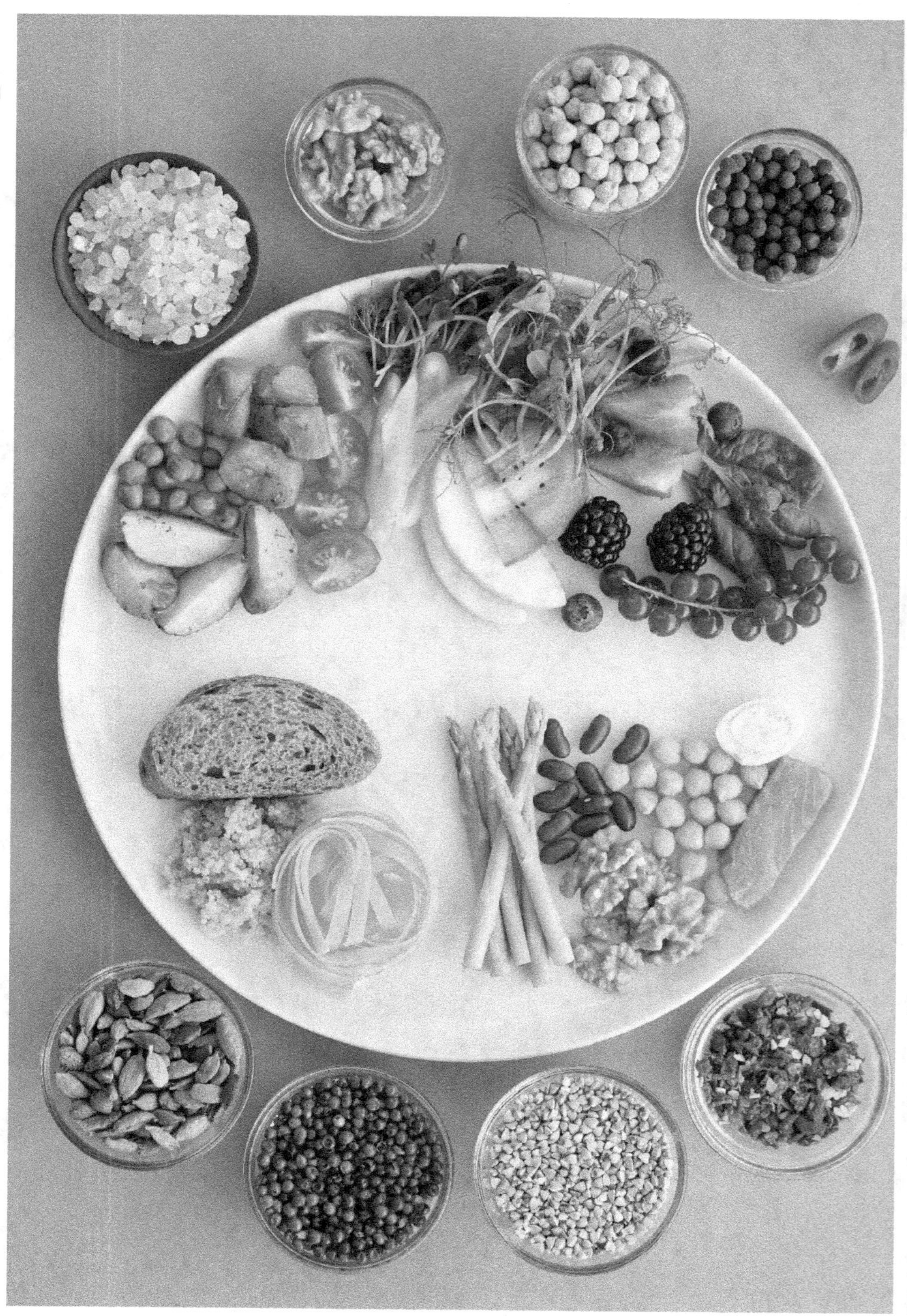

□ 30 Days Plant-Based Diet for Aging □

Are you ready to turn back the clock? Discover the secret to a more young, energetic you with "**30 Days Plant-Based Diet for Aging**". This transforming guide is more than just a diet plan. It's a lifestyle change that uses the power of plant-based nutrition to slow down the aging process and restore your health.

In just 30 days, you'll experience increased energy, better digestion, clearer skin, and a decrease in age-related ailments. The best part? You'll do it all while having delicious, easy-to-prepare meals that will leave you feeling satisfied and fed.

Don't let age define you. Take control of your health and accept the healing power of plants with "**30 Days Plant-Based Diet for Aging**". Start your road to a younger, better you today! □.

Copyright Information

© 2024 **Dr Evelyn James O.K**. All rights reserved.

Overview

30 Days Plant-Based Diet for Aging is a book that helps you adopt a plant-based diet for better health, life, and happiness. The book gives you with:

- A 4-week meal plan that includes breakfast, lunch, dinner, and snacks, as well as buying notes and nutritional information.

- Over 100 easy and delicious recipes that use healthy and plant-based foods, such as fruits, veggies, grains, legumes, nuts, and seeds.

- A thorough guide on how to eat plant-based in different settings, such as family meetings, parties, restaurants, and travel, as well as tips on how to explain your dietary tastes and needs to others.

- A positive and helpful approach on how to develop a healthy and balanced attitude towards food and eating, and how to deal with common issues and concerns, such as body image, weight, hunger, and feelings.

By following the book, you will feel the benefits of eating more veggies and less animals, such as:

- Preventing or controlling chronic diseases, such as diabetes, heart disease, high blood pressure, high cholesterol, and more, by giving your body the nutrients, vitamins, phytochemicals, and fiber that it needs.

- Supporting your healthy aging, by boosting your immune system, digestion, metabolism, memory, and physical function, and by lowering your inflammation, oxidative stress, and risk of cognitive decline, dementia, and Alzheimer's disease.

- Improving your mood, memory, and happiness, by regulating your blood sugar, insulin, and serotonin levels, and by giving you omega-3 fatty acids, tryptophan, and vitamin B12, which can help reduce sadness, anxiety, and stress.

- Increasing your self-esteem, confidence, and happiness, by helping you keep or achieve a healthy weight, lower your blood pressure, and improve your skin, hair, and nails, and by matching your food choices with your values, ethics, and beliefs.

- Enjoying and honoring food and eating, by introducing you to new cuisines, ingredients, dishes, and tastes, by teaching you new skills, techniques, and recipes, and by connecting you with other people, cultures, and feelings.

30 Days Plant-Based Diet for Aging is a book that will inspire and drive you to eat plant-based and help you live longer, better, and health

Introduction

Have you ever thought about the secret to endless youth? The key to energy and vigor that crosses the limits of age? What if I told you that the answer lies not in a magical spring or an elusive elixir, but right in your kitchen? Welcome to "30 Days Plant-Based Diet for Aging", a transformative journey that unravels the power of a plant-based diet in boosting health, life, and well-being.

In a world where we are constantly bombarded with new beauty and health trends, it's easy to forget the basics. The truth is, the secret to a bright and youthful life is not found in expensive creams, hard workout routines, or magic pills, but rather, in the food we consume. Our food plays a pivotal role in our general health and well-being, and a plant-based diet, in particular, has been lauded for its numerous benefits.

This book is not just a guide, but an entrance to a more energetic, healthier, and young you. It's a trip that takes you through the myriad benefits of a plant-based diet, from boosting your energy levels and improving your skin tone to enhancing your immunity and avoiding chronic diseases. It's about knowing the profound effect that our food choices have on our health, our lifespan, and our world.

But this is not just about food. It's about an attitude change. It's about making thoughtful choices that help not just us, but also the world around us. It's about adopting a way of life that is healthy, ethical, and kind. It's about knowing that every meal is a chance to feed our bodies, protect our environment, and contribute to a better and more fair world.

So, are you ready to start on this wonderful journey? Are you ready to discover the changing power of a plant-based diet? Are you ready to open the secret to a better, happier, and more youthful life? If so, then let's get started. Because this is not just a 30-day task. It's the beginning of an ongoing journey towards better health and a better world. Welcome aboard!

The Connection Between Diet and Aging

Aging is a natural process that everyone goes through, but the rate at which we age can be greatly affected by our diet. Here's a deeper look into the link between food and aging:

Nutrient Absorption: As we age, our body's ability to take minerals drops. A diet rich in important nutrients can help prevent this and ensure our bodies get what they need.

Oxidative Stress: Oxidative stress happens when there's a mismatch between the production of free radicals and the body's ability to counteract their harmful effects. Diets high in antioxidants, found in fruits and veggies, can help lower oxidative stress and slow down the aging process.

Inflammation: Chronic inflammation is linked to many age-related illnesses such as arthritis, heart disease, and Alzheimer's. Anti-inflammatory foods like berries, fatty fish, and green leafy vegetables can help control inflammation and possibly slow the aging process.

Telomeres: Telomeres are the protected caps at the end of our chromosomes. Their length is a measure of biological aging, and a diet rich in vitamins and minerals can help keep telomere length.

Gut Health: Our gut health plays an important role in our general health and aging process. A diet high in fiber can support a good gut microbiome, which is linked to longevity.

Caloric Restriction: Some study shows that reducing caloric intake without starvation can extend lives. This is thought to be due to lower metabolic rate and reactive stress.

Healthy Fats: Diets rich in healthy fats, such as the Mediterranean diet, have been linked with life. These diets are high in monounsaturated and polyunsaturated fats, which are good for heart health.

While aging is irreversible, how we age is greatly within our control. A balanced, nutrient-rich diet can go a long way in supporting good aging and life. Remember, it's not only about adding years to our life but life to our years.

Benefits of a plant-based diet for older people

A plant-based diet is a diet that consists of mostly or completely foods produced from plants, such as fruits, veggies, grains, legumes, nuts, and seeds. It may or may not include small amounts of animal products, such as eggs, cheese, fish, or meat. A plant-based diet has many benefits for older adults, such as:

Improved heart health: A plant-based diet can lower the chance of heart disease, high blood pressure, and high cholesterol by reducing the intake of saturated fat and cholesterol from animal products and increasing the intake of fiber, vitamins, and nutrients from plant foods.

Improved mood: A plant-based diet can improve mood and mental well-being by giving adequate amounts of complex carbohydrates, omega-3 fatty acids, vitamin B12, folate, and other nutrients that are necessary for brain function and neurotransmitter release.

Chronic disease prevention and management: A plant-based diet can help prevent and manage some common chronic diseases that affect older adults, such as diabetes, cancer, osteoporosis, and cognitive decline, by modulating blood sugar, inflammation, oxidative stress, hormone levels, and gene expression.

What a plant-based diet is and what things are included and banned

A plant-based diet is a diet that consists of mostly foods produced from plants, such as fruits, veggies, grains, legumes, pulses, nuts, seeds, herbs, and spices. It does not include any animal goods such as meat, fish, cheese, eggs, or honey. A plant-based diet can be healthy, balanced, and varied, as it includes a wide range of foods from different plant sources. Some examples of things that are included and omitted in a plant-based diet are:

Included: fresh, frozen, or canned fruits and vegetables; whole grains such as oats, quinoa, brown rice, and buckwheat; legumes such as beans, lentils, chickpeas, and soy products; nuts and seeds such as almonds, walnuts, sunflower seeds, and chia seeds; plant-based oils such as olive, canola, and coconut oil; plant-based milks, yogurts, cheeses, and butter; herbs and spices such as basil, oregano, turmeric, and ginger; plant-based sweeteners such as maple syrup, agave nectar, and stevia.

Excluded: meat, poultry, fish, and seafood; eggs and dairy products such as milk, cheese, and yogurt; honey and other animal-derived products such as gelatin, lard, and bone broth; refined grains such as white bread, white rice, and white pasta; processed foods such as chips, cookies, cakes, and candy; foods high in refined sugars such as soda, juice, and ice cream; foods high in saturated and trans fats such as butter, margarine, and shortening.

My Family Story

I'm Dr Evelyn James O.K, a certified plant-based nutritionist and coach. I used to pursue an MBA, but I shifted my career path 5 years ago when I discovered the power of plant-based nutrition. Let me tell you how it all began.

My partner had several health issues, such as excessive blood pressure and obesity, high cholesterol, and weariness. He was diagnosed with diabetes and prescribed medication for life. I was unhappy with this outcome, and I sought alternative methods to improve his health. I came across various sources that claimed a plant-based diet could prevent and reverse chronic diseases.

I was intrigued by this possibility, and I decided to test it out. I began to prepare more fruits, vegetables, grains, legumes, nuts, and seeds, and he progressively eliminated animal products from his diet. I also learned how to cook delectable and gratifying plant-based meals, and he relished new flavors and cuisines.

The results were extraordinary. Within a few months, I observed a significant improvement in his blood sugar levels, blood pressure, and vitality levels. He felt happier, more youthful, and more vibrant. He also lost some weight, improved his epidermis, and lowered his cholesterol. His doctor was impressed by his progress, and he reduced his medication dosage. He even said that he might be able to cease taking it completely if he maintained his plant-based lifestyle.

I was astounded by the changes that he experienced, and I wanted to share them with others. I realized that there were many older people who were suffering from similar or worse health problems, and who were searching for a natural and effective method to enhance their well-being. I decided to compose this book to assist them in accomplishing their health goals and enjoying their golden years.

This book is the result of my personal voyage, my investigation, and my passion. I hope that it will inspire you, inform you, and empower you to take control of your health and happiness. I hope that you will join me in this 30-day plant-based challenge, and uncover the amazing benefits of consuming more plants for aging. Thank you for reading, and I wish you all the best.

Part 1: Getting Started with Plant-Based Eating

Chapter 1: How to Plan Your Plant-Based Meals

One of the most important parts of plant-based eating is planning your meals. Planning your meals can help you ensure that you get all the nutrients you need, avoid getting bored or hungry, and save time and money. In this chapter, I'll give you some tips on how to make healthy and satisfying plant-based meals, using the plate method.

What is the plate method?

The plate method is a simple and clear way to plan your plant-based meals. It helps you split your plate into four parts, each representing a different food group. The four food groups are:

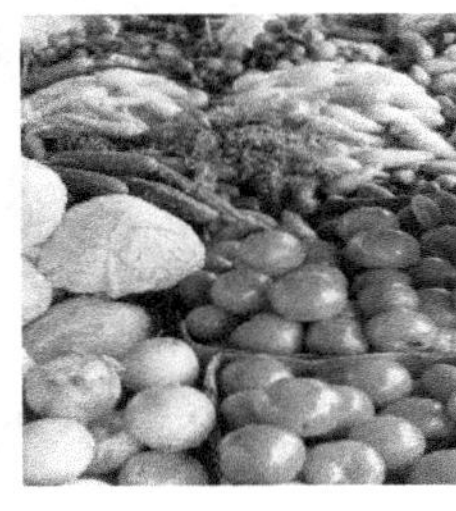

Fruits and vegetables: These are the things that should fill half of your plate. They provide vitamins, minerals, antioxidants, and fiber that support your health and defense.

They also add color, taste, and texture to your food. You can choose fresh, frozen, or canned fruits and veggies, as long as they are not processed with extra sugar, salt, or oil. Try to eat a variety of fruits and veggies, especially dark green, orange, and red ones, as they have more nutrients and phytochemicals.

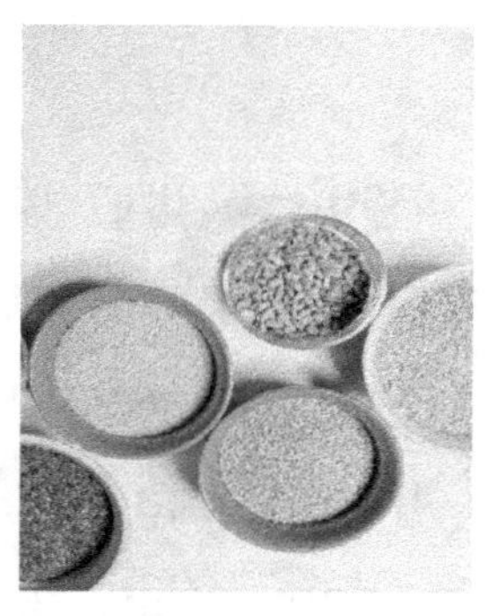

Grains: These are the things that should fill a quarter of your plate. They provide carbs, which are your main source of energy. They also provide fiber, B vitamins, and some minerals. You can choose whole grains, such as oats, quinoa, brown rice, and buckwheat, or refined grains, such as white bread, white rice, and white pasta. However, whole grains are better, as they have more fiber and nutrients, and they keep you fuller for longer. You can also choose gluten-free grains, such as millet, amaranth, and teff if you have gluten intolerance or celiac disease.

Protein: These are the things that should fill the final quarter of your plate. They provide protein, which is important for building and repairing your muscles, bones, skin, and other organs. They also provide iron, zinc, and some other minerals. You can choose plant-based nutrients, such as beans, lentils, chickpeas, soy products, nuts, seeds, and nut butter. You can also choose small amounts of animal-based

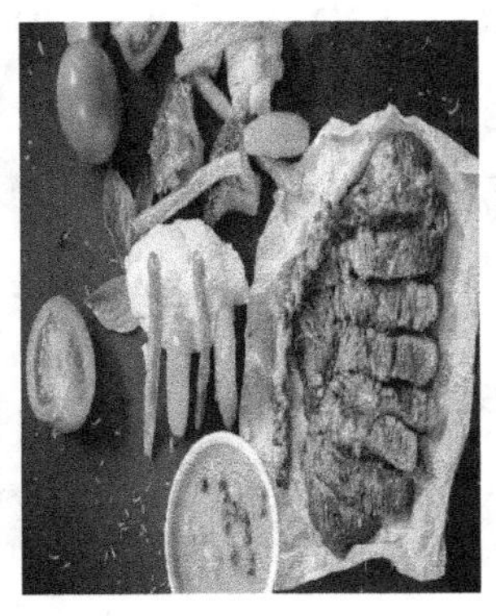

nutrients, such as eggs, dairy, fish, or meat, if you are not completely vegan. However, plant-based proteins are preferred, as they have more fiber and antioxidants, and they are lower in saturated fat and cholesterol.

Healthy fats: These are the foods that should be used carefully, as they provide more calories than the other food groups. They provide fat, which is important for your brain, nerves, hormones, and cell walls. They also provide important fatty acids, such as omega-3 and omega-6, which your body cannot make on its own. You can choose

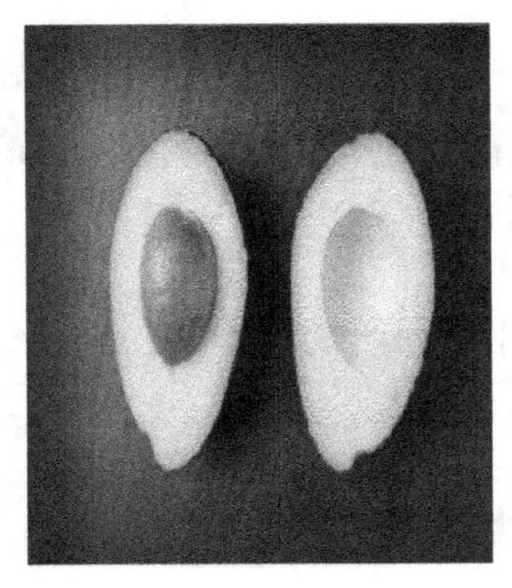

plant-based fats, such as olive, canola, and coconut oil, avocado, nuts, seeds, and nut butter. You can also choose small amounts of animal-based fats, such as butter, cheese, and cream if you are not fully vegan. However, plant-based fats are better, as they have more monounsaturated and polyunsaturated fats, and they are lower in saturated and trans fats.

How to use the plate method

Using the plate method is easy and customizable. You can use it for any meal, whether it is breakfast, lunch, dinner, or snack. You can also use it for any dish, whether it is Asian, Mediterranean, Mexican, or Indian. You can also use it for any food choice, whether it is vegan, vegetarian, gluten-free, or low-carb. Here are some steps to take when using the plate method:

Step 1: Choose a plate that is about 9 inches in diameter. This will allow you to regulate your portion sizes and prevent overeating.

Step 2: Fill half of your plate with fruits and veggies. You can choose raw or cooked, whole or chopped, fresh or frozen, or canned. You can also mix and match different fruits and veggies, such as salad, stir-fry, soup, or shake. You can also add some herbs and spices, such as basil, oregano, turmeric, or ginger, to improve the flavor and health benefits of your fruits and veggies.

Step 3: Fill a quarter of your plate with grains. You can choose whole or refined, cooked or raw, plain or sweetened, or gluten-free. You can also mix and match different grains, such as oatmeal, quinoa, brown rice, or pasta. You can also add some sauces, dressings, or toppings, such as tomato sauce, pesto, or cheese, to improve the taste and texture of your grains.

Step 4: Fill the final quarter of your plate with protein. You can choose plant-based or animal-based, cooked or fresh, plain or spiced, or organic. You can also mix and match different proteins, such as beans, lentils, chickpeas, soy products, nuts, seeds, nut butter, eggs, cheese, fish, or meat. You can also add some seasonings, marinades, or dips, such as soy sauce, barbecue sauce, or hummus, to improve the taste and nutrition of your meats.

Step 5: Add some healthy fats to your plate. You can choose plant-based or animal-based, liquid or solid, plain or spiced, or polished or unrefined. You can also mix and match different fats, such as olive, canola, and coconut oil, avocado, nuts, seeds, nut butter, butter, cheese, and cream. You can also use some cooking methods, such as frying, baking, or sautéing, to add some healthy fats to your foods. However, use them carefully, as they are high in calories and can add up quickly.

Examples of plant-based meals using the plate method

Here are some examples of plant-based meals that you can make using the plate method:

Breakfast: Oatmeal with fresh berries, nuts, and almond milk (fruits and veggies, grains, protein, and good fats)

How to Make for Elderly People

1. Ingredients: Gather your almond milk, oats, and your choice of fresh berries and nuts, preferably unsalted.
2. Cook the oats: In a saucepan, combine one cup of oats with two cups of water. After bringing to a boil, lower the heat to a simmer and cook, stirring now and again, until the oats reach the consistency you prefer, 10 to 20 minutes.
3. As the oatmeal cooks, prepare the toppings by giving the fresh berries a good wash. In case the nuts are too big, you may alternatively cut them into smaller pieces.
4. After the oatmeal is cooked, let it cool for a few minutes before serving. Transfer the oats to a bowl and then generously stir in the almond milk. Add the nuts and fresh berries on top.
5. Have fun: It is now time to savor the food. This well-balanced meal, which includes grains, protein, fruits and vegetables, and healthy fats, is ideal for older adults

Lunch: Vegetable and bean soup with whole wheat bread and hummus (fruits and veggies, grains, protein, and good fats)

How to Make for Elderly People

1. Get the soup ready: Add the chopped celery, carrots, and onions to olive oil and sauté until tender. Add chopped tomatoes, kidney beans, black beans, and chickpeas, along with vegetable broth. Once the beans are soft, simmer them.
2. Get the hummus ready In a food processor, blend chickpeas, tahini, garlic, lemon juice, and olive oil until smooth. Add pepper and salt for seasoning.
3. Accompany the soup with hummus and whole wheat bread on the side.

Dinner: Quinoa and chickpea salad with roasted vegetables and avocado sauce (fruits and vegetables, carbs, protein, and healthy fats)

How to Make for Elderly People

1. Follow the directions on the package to cook the quinoa. Give it time to cool.
2. Add some olive oil, salt, and pepper to the oven and roast whatever veggies you like, such as bell peppers, zucchini, and eggplant.

3. Get the avocado sauce ready. Smoothly puree ripe avocados, garlic, olive oil, and lemon juice in a food processor. Add pepper and salt for seasoning.

4. In a large bowl, combine the chickpeas, roasted veggies, and cooled quinoa. Pour over the avocado sauce and mix well.

Snack: Apple slices with peanut butter and raisins (fruits and veggies, protein, and good fats)

How to Make for Elderly People

1. Cut an apple into slender pieces.
2. On each apple slice, spread a little peanut butter.
3. Dredge the raisins into the peanut butter mixture.

As you can see, using the plate method can help you create healthy and satisfying plant-based meals that are easy to make and delicious to eat. You can also customize them according to your style, choice, and availability. By following the plate method, you can ensure that you get all the nutrients you need while getting the benefits of plant-based eating for age.

how to use leftovers and reuse items.

Using leftovers and reusing items can help you reduce food waste and save time in the kitchen. Here are some suggestions on how to achieve that:

1. Store your leftovers correctly in airtight containers and mark them with the date. Refrigerate them within two hours of cooking and use them within 3 to 4 days, or freeze them for longer keeping. Reheat them properly before eating.

2. Plan your meals ahead and use a shopping list to buy only what you need. Check your fridge, freezer, and closet for things that are about to expire, and use them first. You can also use online tools like **SuperCook** or **BigOven** to find recipes based on the items you have on hand.

3. Transform your leftovers into new meals by adding different spices, sauces, or toppings. For example, you can turn leftover rice into fried rice, leftover pasta into pasta salad, or extra roasted veggies into a frittata. You can also use leftovers as ingredients for sandwiches, wraps, tacos, or quesadillas.

4. Repurpose your ingredients by using different parts of the same food. For example, you can use broccoli stems to make soup, carrot tops to make pesto, or beet

greens to make salad. You can also use vegetable pieces to make stock, fruit peels to make tea, or bread crusts to make croutons.

5. Compost your food waste that cannot be eaten, such as eggshells, coffee grounds, or banana peels. Composting can help you reduce landfill trash and make natural fertilizer for your plants. You can use a compost bin, a worm farm, or a bokashi bucket to compost at home.

sample for 7-day plant-based meal plan with recipes and buying list

To help you eat more plant-based meals, here is a sample 7-day meal plan with recipes and a shopping list. This food plan is based on a 2,000-calorie diet and includes breakfast, lunch, dinner, and snacks. You can change the amounts and calories according to your needs.

Day 1

Breakfast: Overnight oats with almond milk, chia seeds, and fresh berries

steps to make the meals:

1. Combine 1/2 cup of oats, 1/2 cup of almond milk, and 1 tablespoon of chia seeds in a jar.

2. Stir well, cover, and chill overnight.

3. Stir the oats and add fresh berries on top in the morning.

Lunch: Vegetable and bean soup with whole wheat bread and hummus

steps to make the meals:

1. Sauté chopped veggies of your choice (like carrots, celery, and onions) in a pot until cooked.

2. Add a can of beans (drained and rinsed), veggie broth, and spices.

3. Simmer until all the items are well-cooked.

4. Serve with whole wheat bread and hummus.

Dinner: Quinoa and chickpea salad with roasted veggies

steps to make the meals:

1. Cook 1 cup of quinoa according to package directions.

2. In a big bowl, mix cooked quinoa, 1 can of beans (drained and rinsed), and roasted veggies.

3. For the sauce, blend avocado, olive oil, lemon juice, garlic, and spices until smooth.

Snacks: Apple slices with peanut butter and nuts; carrot sticks with ranch dip

steps to make the meals:

1. Apple slices with peanut butter and nuts: Slice an apple
   and serve with a side of peanut butter and a handful of
   nuts.
2. Carrot sticks with ranch dip: Cut carrots into sticks and
   serve with a side of ranch dip.

Day 2

Breakfast: Tofu scramble with spinach, mushrooms, and
cheese; whole wheat toast

steps to make the meals:

1. Sauté spinach and mushrooms in a pan until softened.
2. Crumble tofu into the pan and simmer until heated
   through.
3. Sprinkle with cheese and allow it to soften.
4. Serve with whole wheat crostini.

Lunch: Leftover quinoa and chickpea salad with roasted
veggies and avocado dressing

steps to make the meals:

1. Enjoy the leftover quinoa and chickpea salad from Day
   1's dinner.

Dinner: Black bean and sweet potato tacos with corn tortillas,
salsa, and cilantro

steps to make the meals:

1. Sauté diced sweet potatoes in a pan until softened.

2. Add black beans and sauté until heated through.

3. Spoon the mixture onto maize tortillas.

4. Top with salsa and cilantro.

Snacks: Banana and almond butter drink; popcorn with nutritional yeast

steps to make the meals:

1. Banana and Almond Butter Drink: Blend a banana with a tablespoon of almond butter and a cup of your preferred milk until smooth.

2. Popcorn with Nutritional Yeast: Pop popcorn kernels using your preferred method, then sprinkle with nutritional yeast for a savory flavor.

Day 3

Breakfast: Whole wheat pancakes with maple syrup and walnuts; orange juice

steps to make the meals:

1. Combine baking powder, whole wheat flour, and a small amount of salt.

2. In another bowl, mix milk, an egg, and a bit of vegetable oil.

3. Combine the wet and dry ingredients, then cook on a hot skillet.

4. Serve with maple syrup, peanuts, and a glass of orange juice.

Lunch: Leftover black bean and sweet potato tacos with corn tortillas, salsa, and parsley

steps to make the meals:

1. Enjoy the extra black bean and sweet potato tacos from Day 2's dinner.

Dinner: Lentil and mushroom bolognese with whole wheat spaghetti and veggies

steps to make the meals:

1. Sauté mushrooms in a pan, then add cooked beans and your best pasta sauce.
2. Serve over whole wheat pasta and a side of veggies.

Snacks: Celery sticks with cream cheese and raisins; dark chocolate and almonds

steps to make the meals:

1. Enjoy celery sticks with cream cheese and raisins, and some dark chocolate and nuts.

Day 4

Breakfast: Greek yogurt with nuts and fresh fruit

steps to make the meals:

1. Serve Greek yogurt topped with nuts and fresh fruit.

Lunch: Leftover lentil and mushroom bolognese with whole wheat spaghetti and salad

steps to make the meals:

1. Enjoy the leftover lentil and mushroom bolognese with whole wheat spaghetti and a side salad.

Dinner: Vegetable and tofu stir-fry with brown rice and soy sauce

steps to make the meals:

1. Sauté your favorite veggies and tofu in a pan.
2. Serve with soy sauce on top of brown rice.

Snacks: Edamame with sea salt; oatmeal raisin cookies

steps to make the meals:

1. Enjoy edamame with sea salt and oatmeal raisin cookies.

Day 5

Breakfast: Avocado toast with cooked eggs and cherry tomatoes; green tea

steps to make the meals:

1. Toast a piece of bread and spread avocado mash over it.
2. Top with a cooked egg and cherry tomatoes.
3. Serve with a cup of green tea.

Lunch: Leftover veggie and tofu stir-fry with brown rice and soy sauce

steps to make the meals:

1. Enjoy the leftover veggie and tofu stir-fry with brown rice and soy sauce.

Dinner: Creamy mushroom and spinach rice with parmesan cheese

steps to make the meals:

1. Sauté mushrooms and spinach in a pan.
2. Stir in cooked rice and add a bit of cream.
3. Sprinkle with parmesan cheese before serving.

Snacks: Dried figs and walnuts; kale chips

steps to make the meals:

1. Enjoy dried figs walnuts, and kale chips.

Day 6

Breakfast: Banana and oat muffins with nut butter; milk

steps to make the meals:

1. Mix chopped bananas, oats, eggs, and a bit of nut butter.
2. Bake in a muffin tin until golden.
3. Serve with a glass of milk.

Lunch: Leftover rich mushroom and spinach rice with parmesan cheese

steps to make the meals:

1. Enjoy the reheated creamy mushroom and spinach rice with parmesan cheese.

Dinner: Roasted cauliflower and chickpea soup with naan bread and yogurt

steps to make the meals:

1. Roast broccoli and chickpeas in the oven.
2. Blend with veggie broth until smooth.
3. Serve with naan bread and a spoonful of yogurt.

Snacks: Fresh fruit and cheese; roasted pumpkin seeds

steps to make the meals:

1. Enjoy fresh fruit and cheese, and roasted pumpkin seeds.

Day 7

Breakfast: Veggie omelet with cheese and salsa; whole wheat toast

steps to make the meals:

1. Sauté your best veggies in a pan.
2. Pour whipped eggs over the veggies and cook until set.
3. Sprinkle with cheese and salsa.
4. Serve with whole wheat toast.

Lunch: Leftover roasted cauliflower and chickpea soup with naan bread and yogurt

steps to make the meals:

1. Enjoy the leftover roasted cauliflower and chickpea soup with naan bread and yogurt.

Dinner: Veggie burger with whole wheat bun, lettuce, tomato, onion, and ketchup; oven-baked fries and coleslaw

steps to make the meals:

1. Cook your favorite veggie burger patty.
2. Serve on a whole wheat bun with lettuce, tomato, onion, and ketchup.
3. Serve with oven-baked fries and coleslaw.

Snacks: Strawberry and spinach juice; chips and hummus.

steps to make the meals:

1. Enjoy a strawberry and green juice, and chips with hummus.

Remember to change measure sizes and ingredients as needed to cater to specific dietary needs and tastes. Enjoy your meal preparation!

Shopping List

Fruits: bananas (7), oranges (2), apples (4), berries (2 cups), grapes (2 cups), strawberries (1 cup), lemon (1), lime (1)

Vegetables: spinach (4 cups), mushrooms (2 cups), cherry tomatoes (1 cup), carrots (8), celery (4 stalks), broccoli (1 head), cauliflower (1 head), sweet potatoes (2), onion (4), garlic (1 bulb), ginger (1 piece), cilantro (1 bunch), parsley (1 bunch), lettuce (1 head), tomato (2), avocado (2), kale (4 cups), pumpkin (1 small)

Grains: oats (4 cups), whole wheat bread (1 loaf), quinoa (2 cups), corn tortillas (12), whole wheat spaghetti (1 package), brown rice (2 cups), whole wheat pancakes (8), granola (2 cups), naan bread (4), whole wheat flour (2 cups), whole wheat buns (4)

Legumes: almond milk (4 cups), chia seeds (1/4 cup), hummus (1 cup), chickpeas (3 cans), black beans (2 cans), lentils (2 cups), soy sauce (1/4 cup), tofu (1 block), edamame (2 cups), peanut butter (1/2 cup), almond butter (1/4 cup), cream cheese (1/4 cup), Greek yogurt (2 cups), cheese (2 cups), eggs (12), milk (2 cups), yogurt (2 cups), veggie burgers (4)

Nuts and seeds: walnuts (1/4 cup), nutritional yeast (1/4 cup), almonds (1/4 cup), pistachios (1/4 cup), pumpkin seeds (1/4 cup)

Herbs and spices: salt, pepper, cumin, paprika, chili powder, oregano, basil, thyme, rosemary, turmeric, curry powder, garam masala, cinnamon, nutmeg, vanilla

Other: maple syrup (1/4 cup), salsa (1 cup), ranch dip (1/4 cup), popcorn (4 cups), dark chocolate (1/4 cup), oatmeal raisin cookies (8), dried apricots (1/4 cup), kale chips (2 cups), green tea (4 bags), sea salt (1/4 cup), parmesan cheese (1/4 cup), ketchup (1/4 cup), coleslaw (2 cups), pretzels (2 cups)

Chapter 2: How to Stock Your Plant-Based Pantry

One of the keys to good plant-based living is having a well-stocked pantry. A plant-based pantry is a collection of foods and items that you can use to make delicious and healthy plant-based meals at any time. In this chapter, I'll show you how to stock your plant-based pantry with the important staples, the convenient and healthy products, and the kitchen tools and appliances that can make plant-based cooking easier and more fun.

Essential plant-based staples

The important plant-based staples are the foods and products that you can use as the base for your plant-based meals. They are usually shelf-stable, flexible, and cheap. They can provide you with the macronutrients (carbohydrates, protein, and fat) and the micronutrients (vitamins and minerals) that you need for a healthy plant-based diet. Here are some examples of important plant-based goods and how to use them:

Grains: Grains are the seeds of grasses, such as wheat, rice, oats, and barley. They are rich in carbohydrates, which are your main source of energy. They also provide fiber, B vitamins, and some minerals, such as iron, zinc, and magnesium. You can use grains to make breakfast cereals, breads, soups, snacks, and baked goods. You can also use them as a side dish or a main food, such as rice and beans, quinoa and veggie salad, or oatmeal and fruit. You can choose whole grains, such as brown rice, whole wheat, and oats, or refined grains, such as white rice, white bread, and white pasta. However, whole grains are better, as they have more fiber and nutrients, and they keep you fuller for longer. You can also choose gluten-free grains, such as millet, amaranth, and teff if you have gluten intolerance or celiac disease.

Legumes: Legumes are the seeds of plants that belong to the pea family, such as beans, lentils, chickpeas, and soybeans. They are rich in protein, which is important for building and repairing your muscles, bones, skin, and other organs. They also provide fiber, iron, zinc, folate, and some other nutrients. You can use beans to make soups, stews, sauces, burgers, hummus, and dips. You can also use them as a meat alternative, such as tofu, tempeh, and soy goods. You can choose dried or canned beans, as long as they are not processed with extra sugar, salt, or oil. However, dried beans are preferred, as they are cheaper and have less sodium. You can also sprout your legumes, such as mung beans, alfalfa, and lentils, to improve their digestibility and vitamin content.

Nuts and seeds: Nuts and seeds are the edible kernels of fruits or plants, such as almonds, walnuts, sunflower seeds, and chia seeds. They are rich in fat, which is important for your brain, nerves, hormones, and cell walls. They also provide protein, fiber, omega-3 fatty acids, vitamin E, and some minerals, such as calcium, magnesium, and selenium. You can use nuts and seeds to make nut butter, nut milk, cookies, trail mix, and energy bars. You can also use them as a snack, a topping, or a garnish, such as nuts on oatmeal, sunflower seeds on a salad, or chia seeds on a drink. You can choose raw or roasted nuts and seeds, as long as they are not prepared with extra sugar, salt, or oil. However, raw nuts and seeds are preferred, as they have more enzymes and vitamins.

Spices and herbs: Spices and herbs are the dried or fresh parts of plants that are used to add taste, color, and aroma to your food. They also provide vitamins, phytochemicals, and some minerals, such as iron, manganese, and copper. You can use spices and herbs to make your spice mixes, stews, dressings, and marinades. You can also use them to season your food, such as turmeric on rice, oregano on pizza, or basil on pasta. You can choose whole or ground spices and herbs, as long as they are not made with extra sugar, salt, or preservatives. However, whole spices and herbs are preferred, as they have more taste and freshness. You can also grow your spices and herbs, such as mint, rosemary, and thyme, to have a steady source of fresh and organic ingredients.

Convenient and healthy plant-based items

The handy and healthy plant-based goods are the foods and ingredients that you can buy ready-made or pre-packaged from the store. They are usually refrigerated or frozen, and they have a shorter shelf life than the important plant-based basics. They can provide you with ease, variety, and taste, while still being healthy and nutritious. Here are some examples of handy and healthy plant-based goods and how to use them:

Plant milk: Plant milk is drinks that are made from soaking, mixing, and straining plant-based foods, such as soy, almond, oat, and coconut. They are alternatives to cow's milk, and they can provide calcium, vitamin D, and some other nutrients, based on the type and the preparation. You can use plant milk to make shakes, coffee, tea, and hot chocolate. You can also use them to make breakfast cereals, pancakes, and baked foods. You can choose unsweetened or sweetened plant milks, as long as they are not made with extra sugar, salt, or oil. However, unsweetened plant milks are preferred, as they have fewer calories and sugar. You can also make your plant milk, such as almond milk, oat milk, or rice milk, to save money and avoid chemicals.

Plant yogurts: Plant yogurts are goods that are made from fermenting plant milk, such as soy, almond, coconut, and cashew. They are alternatives to dairy yogurts, and they can provide probiotics, which are helpful bacteria that support your gut health and defense. They can also provide protein, calcium, and some other nutrients, based on the type and the preparation. You can use plant yogurts to make parfaits, dips, and sauces. You can also use them as a snack, a dessert, or a filling, such as soy yogurt with granola and fruit, coconut yogurt with chocolate and nuts, or cashew yogurt with honey and cinnamon. You can choose plain or flavored plant yogurts, as long as they are not made with extra sugar, salt, or oil. However, plain plant yogurts are preferred, as they have less calories and sugar. You can also make your plant yogurts, such as soy yogurt, coconut yogurt, or vegan yogurt, to save money and avoid chemicals.

Plant cheeses: Plant cheeses are goods that are made from growing, aging, or melting plant-based foods, such as cashews, tofu, nutritional yeast, and agar-agar. They are options for dairy cheeses, and they can provide protein, calcium, and some other nutrients, based on the type and the fortification. You can use plant cheeses to make pies, burgers, quesadillas, and nachos. You can also use them as a snack, a dessert, or a treat, such as cashew cheese with crackers and fruit, tofu cheese with jam and bread, or nutritional yeast cheese with popcorn and kale chips. You can choose soft or hard plant cheeses, as long as they are not made with extra sugar, salt, or oil. However, soft plant cheeses are preferred, as they have less calories and fat. You can also make your plant cheeses, such as cashew cheese, tofu cheese, or nutritional yeast cheese, to save money and avoid chemicals.

Tofu and tempeh: Tofu and tempeh are the goods that are made from coagulating and pressing soy milk, or fermenting and binding soybeans, respectively. They are high in protein, iron, calcium, and some other nutrients. They also have a neutral taste and a firm texture, which makes them flexible and adaptable to different cuisines and recipes. You can use tofu and tempeh to make stir-fries, stews, burgers, and nuggets. You can also use them as a meat replacement, such as tofu scramble, tempeh bacon, or tofu steak. You can choose hard or soft tofu, and plain or flavored tempeh, as long as they are not processed with extra sugar, salt, or oil. However, hard tofu and plain tempeh are preferred, as they have more protein and less water. You can also marinate, bake, or fry your tofu and tempeh, to add more taste and structure.

kitchen tools and equipment that can make plant-based cooking easier

Besides the necessary plant-based staples and the handy and healthy plant-based goods, there are some kitchen tools and appliances that can make plant-based cooking easier and more fun. These are the gadgets that can help you prepare, cook, and store your plant-based foods in a faster, easier, and more efficient way. Here are some examples of kitchen tools and gadgets that I suggest and how to use them:

Blender

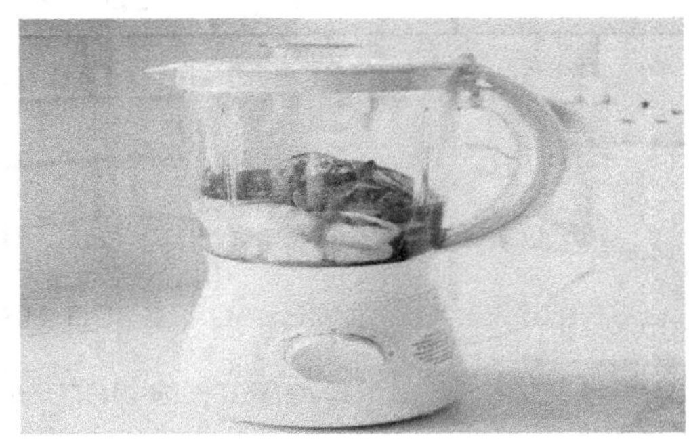

Blender: A blender is a device that can blend, puree, and liquefy different items, such as fruits, veggies, nuts, seeds, and liquids. You can use a blender to make drinks, soups, stews, dressings, nut butter, nut milk, and more. You can choose a high-speed blender, such as a Vitamix or a Blendtec, or a normal blender, such as a Ninja or a Nutribullet. However, a high-speed blender is preferred, as it can handle tougher ingredients, such as ice, frozen fruits, and raw veggies, and create smoother and creamier textures. You can also choose a personal blender, such as a Magic Bullet or an Oster if you want to make single-serve amounts or take your smoothies on the go.

Food processor

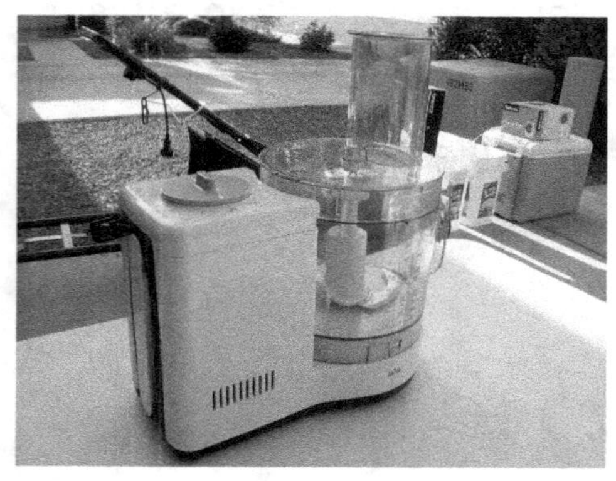

Food processor: A food processor is a device that can chop, slice, shred, grate, and mix different ingredients, such as fruits, veggies, nuts, seeds, and dough. You can use a food processor to make hummus, pesto, chili, cookies, energy bars, and more. You can choose a large-capacity food processor, such as a Cuisinart or a KitchenAid, or a small food processor, such as a Hamilton Beach or a Black+Decker. However, a large-capacity food processor is preferred, as it can handle larger amounts and more functions, such as kneading dough, whipping cream, and emulsifying mayonnaise. You can also choose a food processor with different attachments, such as a blender, a juicer, or a spiralizer, to have more flexibility and ease.

Instant Pot

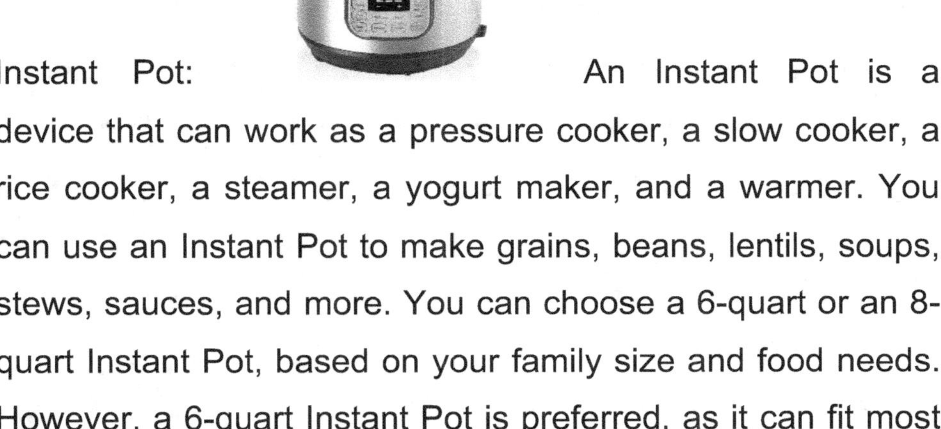

Instant Pot: An Instant Pot is a device that can work as a pressure cooker, a slow cooker, a rice cooker, a steamer, a yogurt maker, and a warmer. You can use an Instant Pot to make grains, beans, lentils, soups, stews, sauces, and more. You can choose a 6-quart or an 8-quart Instant Pot, based on your family size and food needs. However, a 6-quart Instant Pot is preferred, as it can fit most recipes and counter areas. You can also choose an Instant Pot with different features, such as a Duo, a Lux, or an Ultra, to have more choices and settings. You can also use an Instant Pot to make your plant-based yogurt, by following this method.

Air cooker

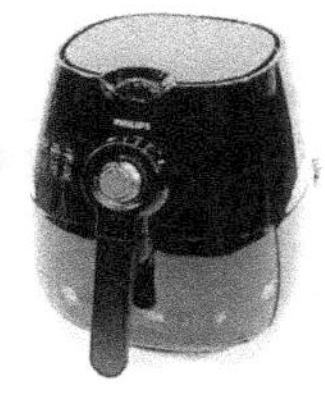

Air fryer: An air fryer is a gadget that can fry, bake, roast, and grill different ingredients, such as potatoes, tofu, tempeh, and veggies, using hot air and little or no oil. You can use an air fryer to make crispy and tasty plant-based meals, such as fries, nuggets, burgers, and chips. You can choose a basket-style or an oven-style air fryer, based on your taste and space. However, an oven-style air fryer is preferred, as it can fit more food and have more functions, such as toasting, broiling, and drying. You can also choose an air fryer with different features, such as a Cosori, a Ninja, or a Breville, to have more choices and settings. You can also use an air fryer to make your plant-based cheese.

Mason jar

Mason jars: Mason jars are glass containers that have a metal lid and a metal ring that can seal the jar tightly. You can use mason jars to store your plant-based foods, such as salads, soups, sauces, dressings, nut butter, nut milk, and more. You can choose different sizes and shapes of mason jars, based on your wants and preferences. However, wide-mouth mason jars are preferred,

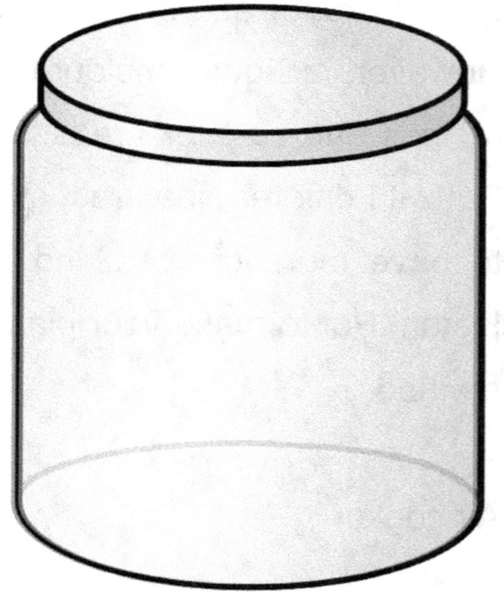

as they are easier to fill and clean. You can also choose mason jars with different lids, such as plastic, bamboo, or silicone, to have more sturdiness and ease. You can also use mason jars to make your plant-based sprouts.

These are some of the kitchen tools and appliances that can make plant-based cooking easier and more enjoyable.

Chapter 3: How to Transition to Plant-Based Eating

Transitioning to plant-based eating can be a rewarding and enjoyable experience, but it can also come with some difficulties and hurdles. In this chapter, I'll address some of the usual problems that you may face when adopting a plant-based diet, and I'll offer some strategies and answers to overcome them. I'll also encourage you to start gradually and try different foods and recipes, and I'll stress the value of listening to your body and making adjustments as required.

Common obstacles and hurdles to plant-based eating

Here are some of the usual hurdles and barriers that you may face when switching to plant-based eating, and <u>some tips on how to deal with them:</u>

Social pressure: You may face some pushback or criticism from your family, friends, or co-workers, who may not understand or support your choice to eat more plants. They may question your goals, your nutrition, or your taste, and they may try to convince you to eat animal products or mock you for your choices. You may also feel separated or ignored in social settings, such as family gatherings, parties, restaurants, or travel, where plant-based choices may be limited or unavailable.

- **How to overcome it:** The best way to deal with social pressure is to be strong, polite, and positive about your plant-based lifestyle. You can explain your reasons and benefits for eating more veggies, without being judgmental or angry. You can also educate yourself and others about the health, environmental, and ethical sides of plant-based eating, by sharing facts, tools, and stories. You can also find support and community from other plant-based eaters, either online or offline, who can relate to your difficulties and share your achievements. You can also plan ahead and prepare for social settings, by bringing your food, checking menus, asking questions, or suggesting plant-based places.

Cravings: You may crave some animal products or processed foods that you used to eat, such as cheese, eggs, bacon, chocolate, or ice cream. You may miss the taste, texture, or warmth that these foods provide, and you may feel tempted to give in to your cravings. You may also experience some withdrawal effects, such as headaches, fatigue, or mood swings, as your body changes to the new food.

- **How to overcome it:** The best way to deal with urges is to recognize them, understand them, and healthily satisfy them. You can recognize your needs, without judging or shaming yourself. You can understand your cravings, by finding the triggers, feelings, or needs that cause them. You can fill your cravings, by finding plant-based options or substitutes that can mimic or replace the foods you crave, such as plant-based cheeses, eggs, bacon, chocolate, or ice cream. You can also separate yourself from your cravings, by participating in other activities, such as exercise, meditation, or hobbies. You can also be patient and determined, as your cravings will likely lessen or disappear over time, as your taste buds and habits change.

Cost: You may think that eating more plants is expensive, especially if you buy organic, fresh, or specialty goods, such as fruits, veggies, nuts, seeds, or plant-based meats. You may also think that eating more veggies is wasteful, especially if you throw away spoiled or wasted food. You may also think that eating more plants is inconvenient, especially if you have to shop more frequently or drive farther to find plant-based choices.

- **How to overcome it:** The best way to deal with cost is to be smart, clever, and sustainable about your plant-based shopping and cooking. You can be smart, by planning your meals ahead, using a shopping list, and getting only what you need. You can also be smart, by comparing prices, looking for deals, coupons, or discounts, and buying in bulk, season, or frozen. You can also be sustainable, by using leftovers, reusing ingredients, and composting food waste. You can also save money and time, by making your plant-based goods, such as plant milks, yogurts, cheeses, tofu, tempeh, or seitan.

Strategies and solutions to overcome these challenges

In addition to the tips I gave you for dealing with the usual challenges and hurdles to plant-based eating, here are some more **strategies and solutions** that can help you beat them and succeed in your plant-based journey:

Find support: Having a helpful network of people who share your values, goals, and experiences can make a big difference in your plant-based transition. You can find support from your family, friends, or co-workers, who can encourage you, push you, and join you in your plant-based meals. You can also find help from other plant-based eaters, either online or offline, who can offer you advice, comments, and inspiration. You can join online groups, such as [VeggieBoards], [HappyCow], or [Reddit], where you can chat, ask questions, and share stories with other plant-based eaters. You can also join offline groups, such as [Meetup], [VegFest], or [PlantPure], where you can meet, connect, and learn from other plant-based eaters in your area.

Set goals: Having clear and reasonable goals can help you stay focused, committed, and accountable in your plant-based shift. You can set short-term and long-term goals, such as eating more veggies for a week, a month, or a year, or eating fewer animal products for a day, a week, or a month. You can also set specific and measured goals, such as eating at least five servings of fruits and veggies a day or cutting your intake of saturated fat by 10%. You can also set personal and important goals, such as bettering your health, saving the environment, or agreeing with your ethics.

Track success: Tracking your progress can help you track your achievements, obstacles, and changes in your plant-based transition. You can track your progress using different ways, such as keeping a food log, using an app, or taking photos. You can also track your progress using different markers, such as your weight, your blood pressure, your cholesterol, or your energy levels. You can also track your progress using different schedules, such as daily, weekly, or monthly. Tracking your progress can help you celebrate your wins, find your areas of improvement, and change your goals and strategies as needed.

Start gradually: Transitioning to plant-based eating does not have to be an all-or-nothing method. You can start gradually and make small and regular changes in your diet, such as adding more fruits and veggies to your meals, replacing some animal products with plant-based alternatives, or having one or two plant-based days a week. Starting gradually can help you ease into the new diet, avoid overloading yourself, and build your confidence and skills.

Experiment with different foods and recipes: Transitioning to plant-based eating can be a fun and exciting chance to try new foods and recipes. You can explore different foods and recipes, such as trying new countries, ingredients, dishes, or tastes. You can also try different ways of making and cooking your foods, such as roasting, baking, or sautéing. Experimenting with different foods and recipes can help you discover new tastes, textures, and combinations, and make your plant-based meals more fun and rewarding.

Listen to your body: Transitioning to plant-based eating can have different effects on your body, depending on your individual needs, tastes, and reactions. You can listen to your body and make changes as needed, such as increasing or decreasing your portions, calories, or nutrients, adding or removing certain foods or ingredients, or changing your eating frequency or time. Listening to your body can help you find the ideal balance and unity for your health and well-being.

These are some of the strategies and solutions that I suggest you use to beat the difficulties and barriers to plant-based eating. By following these tips, you can make your plant-based shift easier, faster, and more successful.

I hope you found this part helpful and useful. I want to encourage you to start gradually and play with different foods and recipes as you move to plant-based eating. You don't have to make drastic or sudden changes, but rather small and regular ones that suit your wants and tastes. You can also have fun and be creative with your plant-based meals, by trying new cuisines, ingredients, dishes, or tastes. You may be surprised by how delicious and satisfying plant-based eating can be.

I also want to stress the value of listening to your body and making adjustments as needed as you transition to plant-based eating. Your body may respond differently to the new diet, based on your factors, such as your age, health, exercise level, and metabolism. You may need to increase or decrease your portions, calories, or nutrients, add or remove certain foods or ingredients, or change your eating regularly or time. You can also watch your health markers, such as your weight, blood pressure, cholesterol, or blood sugar, to see how your plant-based diet changes them. Listening to your body can help you find the ideal balance and unity for your health and well-being.

Part 2: Plant-Based Eating for Aging Well

Chapter 4: How to Meet Your Nutritional Needs on a Plant-Based Diet

In this chapter, I'll explain how to meet your nutritional requirements on a plant-based diet, and how this can support your healthy aging. I'll also emphasize some essential nutrients that older adults may need more of, and how to get them from plant-based sources. I'll also discuss the pros and cons of taking supplements, and when they may be necessary.

The significance of macronutrients and micronutrients in healthful aging

Macronutrients and micronutrients are the two primary types of nutrients that your body requires to function correctly. Macronutrients are the nutrients that provide sustenance and structure to your body, such as protein, carbohydrates, and lipids. Micronutrients are the nutrients that regulate your body's processes and protect your cells from injury, such as vitamins and minerals.

Both macronutrients and micronutrients play essential roles in supporting your healthy aging, as they help you maintain your muscle mass, bone density, immune system, cognitive function, and overall well-being. However, as you age, your nutritional requirements may alter, due to factors such as reduced appetite, decreased absorption, increased inflammation, or medication interactions. Therefore, you may need to modify your intake of certain nutrients, to ensure that you get enough of them, and avoid deficiencies or excesses.

Key nutrients that older adults may need more of

Here are some of the key nutrients that older adults may need more of, and <u>why they are important for your health:</u>

Calcium: Calcium is a mineral that is essential for constructing and maintaining strong bones and teeth. It also assists with muscle contraction, nerve transmission, blood coagulation, and hormone secretion. As you age, your bone density may decline, increasing your risk of osteoporosis and fractures. Therefore, you may need more calcium to prevent bone loss and support your skeletal health. The recommended daily dose of calcium for people over 50 is 1200 mg.

Vitamin D: Vitamin D is a fat-soluble vitamin that helps your body absorb and use calcium. It also assists with immune function, inflammation, mood, and cognitive function. As you age, your epidermis may produce less vitamin D from sunlight exposure, and your kidneys may convert less vitamin D to its active form. Therefore, you may need more vitamin D to prevent deficiency and support your bone and overall health. The recommended daily intake of vitamin D for adults over 50 is 15 mcg (600 IU).

Vitamin B12: Vitamin B12 is a water-soluble vitamin that is involved in the production of red blood cells, DNA, and nerve function. It also assists with energy metabolism, brain function, and mood. As you age, your stomach may produce less acid, which is needed to liberate vitamin B12 from food. Therefore, you may need more vitamin B12 to prevent deficiency and support your blood and nervous system health. The recommended daily intake of vitamin B12 for adults over 50 is 2.4 mcg.

Iron: Iron is a mineral that is essential for transporting oxygen in your blood, and for producing hemoglobin, the protein that transports oxygen. It also assists with energy production, immune function, and wound healing. As you age, you may lose more iron due to hemorrhage, inflammation, or medication use. Therefore, you may need more iron to prevent anemia and support your oxygen delivery and overall health. The recommended daily intake of iron for adults over 50 is 8 milligrams for men and 8 mg for women.

Zinc: Zinc is a mineral that is involved in many enzymatic reactions in your body, such as protein synthesis, DNA synthesis, and wound healing. It also assists with immune function, taste perception, and skin health. As you age, your zinc absorption may decrease, and your zinc losses may increase due to infection, stress, or medication use. Therefore, you may need more zinc to prevent deficiency and support your immune and overall health. The recommended daily intake of zinc for adults over 50 is 11 milligrams for men and 8 mg for women.

Plant-based sources of essential nutrients and how to include them in your diet

You can get most of the essential nutrients that you need from plant-based sources, as long as you consume a varied and balanced diet. Here are some examples of plant-based sources of essential nutrients and how to include them in your diet:

Calcium: You can get calcium from plant-based foods such as verdant green vegetables (such as kale, collard greens, and bok choy), broccoli, tofu, tempeh, almonds, sesame seeds, chia seeds, fortified plant milk, yogurts, and cheeses. You can include these foods in your meals and treats, such as adding kale to your smoothie, broccoli to your stir-fry, tofu to your curry, almonds to your oatmeal, sesame seeds to your salad, chia seeds to your pudding, or fortified plant milk to your coffee.

Vitamin D: You can get vitamin D from plant-based foods such as mushrooms, fortified plant milks, yogurts, and cereals. You can also get vitamin D from sunlight exposure, but this may vary depending on your skin color, location, season, and time of day. You can include these foods in your meals and treats, such as adding mushrooms to your omelet, fortified plant milk to your cereal, yogurt to your parfait, or cereal to your trail mix. You can also attempt to get some sunlight exposure every day, but be cautious not to burn your skin or damage your eyes.

Vitamin B12: You can get vitamin B12 from plant-based foods such as fortified plant milks, yogurts, cheeses, cereals, nutritional yeast, and supplements. You can include these foods in your meals and nibbles, such as adding fortified plant milk to your smoothie, yogurt to your granola, cheese to your sandwich, cereal to your muffin, nutritional yeast to your popcorn, or taking a supplement as directed by your doctor or dietitian.

Iron: You can get iron from plant-based foods such as legumes, lentils, chickpeas, soy products, nuts, seeds, dried fruits, whole cereals, and dark green leafy vegetables. You can include these foods in your meals and snacks, such as adding beans to your soup, lentils to your salad, chickpeas to your hummus, soy products to your stir-fry, nuts to your trail mix, seeds to your bread, dried fruits to your cookies, whole grains to your pilaf, or dark green leafy vegetables to your smoothie. You can also enhance your iron assimilation by consuming foods rich in vitamin C, such as citrus fruits, berries, tomatoes, peppers, or broccoli, along with your iron-rich foods.

Zinc: You can get zinc from plant-based foods such as legumes, lentils, chickpeas, soy products, nuts, seeds, whole grains, and fungi. You can include these foods in your meals and treats, such as adding legumes to your chili, lentils to your burger, chickpeas to your falafel, soy products to your tacos, almonds to your brownies, seeds to your crackers, whole grains to your pancakes, or mushrooms to your pizza. You can also enhance your zinc absorption by soaking, sprouting, or fermenting your plant-based foods, or by consuming foods rich in sulfur, such as garlic, onion, or scallions, along with your zinc-rich foods.

The merits and cons of consuming supplements and when they may be necessary

Taking supplements can be a way to ensure that you get enough of the key nutrients that you need, particularly if your diet is not varied or balanced, or if you have certain medical conditions or medications that impact your nutrient absorption or metabolism. However, consuming supplements can also have some drawbacks, such as cost, quality, safety, or interactions. Therefore, you should evaluate the pros and cons of taking supplements, and consult with your doctor or dietitian before taking them. Here are some of the pros and cons of consuming supplements and when they may be necessary:

Pros: Taking supplements can help you prevent or treat nutrient deficiencies, enhance your health outcomes, and reduce your risk of chronic diseases. Taking supplements can also be convenient, simple, and consistent, as you can take them at any time and place, and you don't have to stress about cooking or preparing your food. Taking supplements can also be customized, as you can choose the type, dose, and form of the supplement that suits your requirements and preferences.

Cons: Taking supplements can be expensive, as they can add up to your monthly budget, and they may not be covered by your insurance or health plan. Taking supplements can also be dubious, as they may not be regulated, tested, or standardized, and they may contain contaminants, additives, or fillers. Taking supplements can also be hazardous, as they may have side effects, adverse reactions, or interactions with your other medications, supplements, or foods. Taking supplements can also be misleading, as they may not be effective, necessary, or appropriate for your condition, and they may not replace a balanced and varied diet.

When they may be necessary: Taking supplements may be necessary if you have a diagnosed or suspected nutrient deficiency, such as insufficient levels of vitamin D, vitamin B12, iron, or zinc, and if your diet is not sufficient to meet your requirements. Taking supplements may also be necessary if you have a medical condition or medication that impacts your nutrient assimilation or metabolism, such as celiac disease, Crohn's disease, gastric bypass surgery, or metformin. Taking supplements may also be necessary if you have a higher nutrient requirement or a reduced nutrient consumption, such as during pregnancy, lactation, menopause, or aging. Taking supplements may also be necessary if you have a specific health objective or concern, such as enhancing your bone health, immune function, or cognitive function, and if your diet is not optimal to support it.

Chapter 5: How to Boost Your Immune System with Plant-Based Foods

In this chapter, I'll show you how to strengthen your immune system with plant-based nutrients, and how this can support your healthy aging. I'll also describe how the immune system functions and how it changes with age, identify some factors that can impair or strengthen the immune system, and share some immune-boosting recipes that you can enjoy.

How the immune system functions and how it changes with age

The immune system is a complex network of cells, tissues, and organs that protect your body from detrimental invaders, such as bacteria, viruses, fungi, and parasites. The immune system consists of two primary parts: the innate immune system and the adaptive immune system. The innate immune system is the first line of defense, and it responds rapidly and extensively to any foreign substance. The innate immune system includes physical barriers, such as your epidermis and mucous membranes, and cells, such as macrophages, neutrophils, and natural killer cells. The adaptive immune system is the second line of defense, and it responds specifically and selectively to the invaders that have been recognized by the innate immune system. The adaptive immune system comprises cells, such as B cells and T cells, and molecules, such as antibodies and cytokines.

As you age, your immune system may decline, making you more susceptible to infections, inflammation, and chronic diseases. This decline is termed immunosenescence, and it can affect both the innate and the adaptive immune system. Some of the changes that occur in your immune system as you age are:

1. Reduced production and function of immune cells, such as macrophages, neutrophils, natural killer cells, B cells, and T cells.

2. Reduced diversity and memory of immune cells, making them less able to recognize and respond to new or recurring invaders.

3. Reduced production and quality of antibodies, rendering them less effective in neutralizing and eliminating the invaders.

4. Increased production and activity of pro-inflammatory cytokines, make you more prone to inflammation and tissue injury.

5. Reduced communication and coordination between the innate and the adaptive immune system, rendering them less efficient and harmonious.

These alterations can make you more vulnerable to infections, such as colds, flu, pneumonia, and urinary tract infections. They can also make you more likely to develop chronic diseases, such as diabetes, cardiovascular disease, cancer, and autoimmune disorders. They can also make you less responsive to vaccines, which are designed to stimulate your immune system and protect you from certain diseases. Therefore, it is essential to take care of your immune system as you age and to strengthen it with plant-based foods that can help enhance its function and performance.

Factors that can impair or enhance the immune system

Besides aging, there are other factors that can influence your immune system, either positively or negatively. Some of the factors that can impair your immune system are:

Stress: Stress is a condition of mental or emotional strain or tension that can result from challenging or demanding situations. Stress can prompt the release of hormones, such as cortisol and adrenaline, that can suppress your immune system and make you more susceptible to infections and inflammation. Stress can also impact your mood, sleep, appetite, and behavior, which can further compromise your immune health.

Sleep: Sleep is a state of rest and recuperation that can affect your physical and mental health. Sleep can help regulate your immune system and enhance its function and performance. Sleep can also help reduce inflammation and oxidative stress, which can damage your cells and tissues. Sleep deprivation, on the other hand, can impair your immune system and make you more prone to infections and chronic diseases. Sleep deprivation can also affect your temperament, cognition, memory, and learning, which can impact your immune health.

Exercise: Exercise is a physical activity that can enhance your health and well-being. Exercise can help stimulate your immune system and increase its activity and efficiency. Exercise can also help reduce inflammation, oxidative stress, and blood pressure, which can benefit your immune health. Exercise can also help enhance your mood, sleep, and metabolism, which can support your immune health. However, too much or too intense exercise can have the opposite effect, and impair your immune system and make you more vulnerable to infections and inflammation. Therefore, it is essential to exercise moderately and regularly and to rest and recuperate adequately.

Diet: Diet is the food and drink that you ingest on a daily basis. Diet can have a significant impact on your immune system, as it can provide or deprive you of the nutrients that your immune system requires to function effectively. A healthy and balanced diet can help nourish your immune system and enhance its function and performance. A healthy and balanced diet can also help prevent or manage chronic diseases, such as diabetes, cardiovascular disease, and cancer, that can impair your immune system. A poor and unbalanced diet, on the other hand, can damage your immune system and make you more susceptible to infections and inflammation. A poor and unbalanced diet can also cause or worsen chronic diseases, such as obesity, hypertension, and dyslipidemia, that can compromise your immune health.

<u>Some of the factors that can strengthen your immune system are:</u>

Relaxation: Relaxation is a state of calmness and harmony that can result from engaging in activities that make you feel joyful and comfortable. Relaxation can help reduce stress and its negative effects on your immune system. Relaxation can also help improve your mood, sleep, and appetite, which can benefit your immune health. Some of the activities that can help you calm down are meditation, yoga, breathing exercises, massage, music, reading, or pastimes.

Hygiene: Hygiene is the practice of keeping yourself and your surroundings clean and free of pathogens and grime. Hygiene can help prevent or reduce exposure to detrimental invaders that can cause infections and diseases. Hygiene can also help protect your immune system and enhance its function and performance. Some of the practices that can help you maintain good sanitation are washing your hands, brushing your teeth, bathing, cleaning your clothing, and disinfecting your surfaces.

Vaccination: Vaccination is the process of introducing an attenuated or slain form of an invader into your body, to stimulate your immune system and protect you from the disease that the invader causes. Vaccination can help enhance your immune system and increase its memory and diversity. Vaccination can also help prevent or reduce the severity of infections and diseases, such as measles, mumps, rubella, tetanus, hepatitis, and influenza. Vaccination can also help protect others, particularly those who are more vulnerable, such as infants, elderly, or immunocompromised, from getting infected and ill. Therefore, it is crucial to observe the recommended vaccination schedule and get the appropriate vaccines for your age and condition.

Plant-based foods: Plant-based foods are foods that are derived from plants, such as fruits, vegetables, cereals, legumes, nuts, and seeds. Plant-based foods can help enhance your immune system and support your healthy aging, as they can provide you with the macronutrients and micronutrients that your immune system requires to function properly. Plant-based foods can also provide you with antioxidants, phytochemicals, and fiber, that can help reduce inflammation, oxidative stress, and blood sugar, which can benefit your immune health. Plant-based diets can also help prevent or manage chronic diseases, such as diabetes, cardiovascular disease, and cancer, that can impair your immune system. Therefore, it is recommended to consume more plant-based foods and fewer animal products, as part of a healthy and balanced diet.

plant-based nutrients that can help enhance the immune

Some plant-based nutrients that can help enhance the immune system are:

Fruit

- Fruits: Fruits are rich in vitamin C, which is essential for the production and function of immune cells. Vitamin C also has antioxidant and anti-inflammatory properties, which can help protect your cells from injury and infection. Some fruits that are high in vitamin C are citrus fruits, such as oranges, grapefruits, lemons, and limes, berries, such as strawberries, blueberries, raspberries, and cranberries, and kiwis, papayas, and pineapples.

Vegetable

- Vegetables: Vegetables are also abundant in vitamin C, as well as other vitamins, minerals, and phytochemicals that can support your immune system. Some vegetables that are high in vitamin C are bell peppers, broccoli, cauliflower, Brussels sprouts, and cabbage. Other vegetables that can enhance your immunity are leafy greens, such as spinach, kale, and collard greens, which are high in folate, iron, and vitamin K, and mushrooms, which are high in vitamin D, selenium, and beta-glucans.

Herbs and spices:

- Herbs and spices: Herbs and spices can contribute flavor and aroma to your food, as well as immune-boosting benefits. Some herbs and seasonings that can help enhance your immune system are garlic, ginger, turmeric, cinnamon, oregano, rosemary, and thyme. Garlic and ginger have antibacterial, antiviral, and anti-inflammatory properties, which can help ward off infections and reduce inflammation. Turmeric and cinnamon have antioxidant and anti-inflammatory properties, which can help protect your cells from oxidative stress and inflammation. Oregano, rosemary, and thyme have antimicrobial and antifungal properties, which can help prevent or treat fungal and bacterial infections.

<u>Some immune-boosting recipes that you can attempt are:</u>

Citrus Berry Smoothie: This smoothie is a delectable and refreshing way to start your day with a dose of vitamin C and antioxidants. To prepare it, you will need 1 cup of orange juice, 1/2 cup of frozen mixed berries, 1/4 cup of plain or vanilla plant-based yogurt, and 1 tablespoon of hemp seeds. Blend all the ingredients until smooth and enjoy.

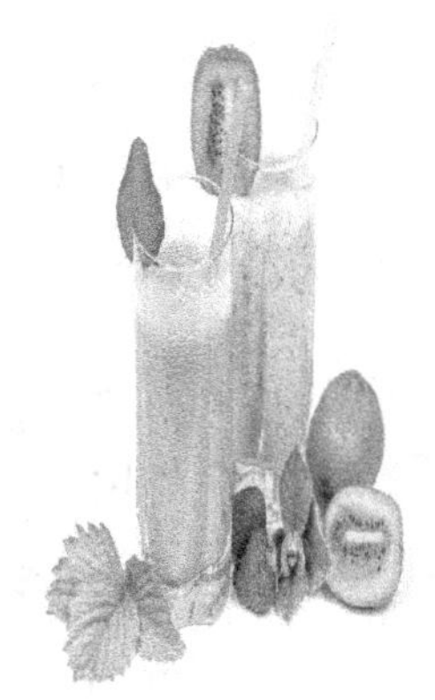

Broccoli Broccoli and Red Lentil Soup: This soup is a hearty and satisfying entrée that is rich in protein, fiber, vitamin C, and iron. To make it, you will need 1 tablespoon of olive oil, 1 onion, chopped, 4 cloves of garlic, minced, 1 teaspoon of turmeric, 1/4 teaspoon of salt, 4 cups of vegetable broth, 1 cup of red lentils, rinsed and drained, and 4 cups of broccoli florets. Heat the oil in a large kettle over medium-high heat and sauté the onion and garlic for about 15 minutes, stirring intermittently, until soft and golden. Add the turmeric and salt and simmer for another minute, stirring. Add the broth and beans and bring to a simmer. Reduce the heat

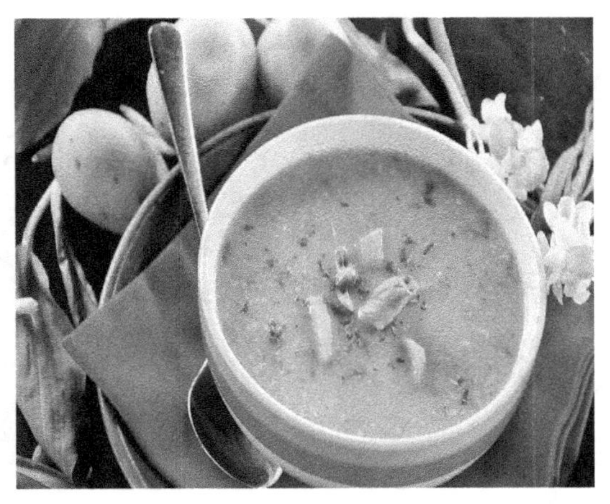

and simmer for about 20 minutes, until the legumes are tender. Add the broccoli and sauté for another 10 minutes, until the broccoli is vibrant green and crisp-tender. You can savor the broth as it is, or blend it for a creamier texture.

Kale

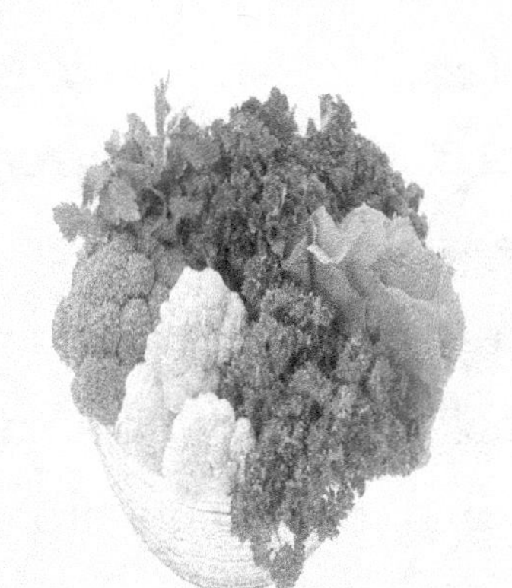

Kale and Quinoa Salad: This salad is a light and nutritious dish that is full of folate, iron, vitamin K, and zinc. To make it, you will need 2 cups of cooked quinoa, 4 cups of minced kale, 1/4 cup of chopped almonds, 1/4 cup of dried cranberries, 2 tablespoons of lemon juice, 2 tablespoons of olive oil, 1 teaspoon of maple syrup, 1/4 teaspoon of salt, and 1/4 teaspoon of black pepper. In a large basin, combine the quinoa, kale, almonds, and cranberries. In a small basin, whisk the lemon juice, olive oil, maple syrup, salt, and pepper. Drizzle the dressing over the salad and swirl to combine. You can savor the salad as a primary or a side dish.

Chapter 6: How to Prevent and Manage Chronic Diseases with Plant-Based Foods

In this chapter, I'll show you how a plant-based diet can help avoid and treat some common chronic diseases that affect older adults, such as diabetes, heart disease, high blood pressure, high cholesterol, and more. I'll also provide scientific proof and studies that support the link between plant-based eating and chronic disease prevention and control. I'll also give you some practical tips and advice on how to follow a plant-based diet for specific health problems, and I'll share some success stories and comments from people who have improved their health with plant-based eating.

How a plant-based diet can help avoid and control chronic diseases

A plant-based diet is a diet that emphasizes foods that are derived from plants, such as fruits, veggies, grains, legumes, nuts, and seeds and minimizes or avoids foods that are derived from animals, such as meat, dairy, eggs, and fish. A plant-based diet can help avoid and control chronic diseases, as it can provide you with the following benefits:

Lower blood sugar: A plant-based diet can help lower your blood sugar, as it can provide you with complex carbohydrates, fiber, and vitamins, that can help control your insulin and glucose levels. A plant-based diet can also help avoid or lessen insulin resistance, which is a condition where your cells become less responsive to insulin, and your blood sugar rises. A plant-based diet can also help avoid or manage diabetes, which is an illness where your blood sugar is too high, and can cause complications, such as nerve damage, kidney damage, eye damage, and heart disease.

Lower blood pressure: A plant-based diet can help lower your blood pressure, as it can provide you with potassium, magnesium, calcium, and nitric oxide, which can help relax your blood vessels and reduce your blood pressure. A plant-based diet can also help avoid or decrease sodium intake, which is a mineral that can increase your blood pressure. A plant-based diet can also help avoid or manage hypertension, which is a disease where your blood pressure is too high, and can cause damage to your heart, brain, kidneys, and eyes.

Lower cholesterol: A plant-based diet can help lower your cholesterol, as it can provide you with soluble fiber, phytosterols, and unsaturated fats, that can help reduce your LDL (bad) cholesterol and raise your HDL (good) cholesterol. A plant-based diet can also help avoid or reduce saturated fat and trans fat intake, which are types of fat that can raise your LDL cholesterol and lower your HDL cholesterol. A plant-based diet can also help avoid or manage dyslipidemia, which is a situation where your cholesterol levels are abnormal and can increase your risk of heart disease and stroke.

Lower inflammation: A plant-based diet can help lower your inflammation, as it can provide you with vitamins, phytochemicals, and omega-3 fatty acids that can help reduce your reactive stress and inflammation. Oxidative stress and inflammation are processes where your cells are harmed by free radicals, which are unstable chemicals that can cause harm to your DNA, proteins, and membranes. A plant-based diet can also help prevent or decrease animal protein and animal fat intake, which are sources of arachidonic acid, which is a type of omega-6 fatty acid that can raise oxidative stress and inflammation. A plant-based diet can also help avoid or treat chronic diseases that are linked with inflammation, such as arthritis, asthma, allergies, and autoimmune disorders.

Scientific proof and studies that show the link between plant-based eating and chronic illness prevention and control

There is a growing amount of scientific data and studies that support the link between plant-based eating and chronic disease prevention and management. **Here are some of the most important and current ones:**

1. A meta-analysis of 9 randomized controlled studies involving 307 participants showed that a plant-based diet can significantly lower blood sugar, blood pressure, and cholesterol, compared to a control diet, in people with type 2 diabetes.

2. A prospective cohort study of 15,428 people from the Adventist Health Study-2 found that a plant-based diet can lower the chance of hypertension by 34%, compared to a non-vegetarian diet, after adjusting for confounding factors.

3. A randomized controlled study of 198 participants with coronary artery disease found that a plant-based diet can lower the frequency of angina (chest pain) by 91%, compared to a control diet, after 12 weeks of intervention.

4. A thorough review and meta-analysis of 40 studies covering 12,915 people found that a plant-based diet

can lower the levels of C-reactive protein (CRP), which is a marker of inflammation, by 0.55 mg/L, compared to a control diet.

Tips and advice on how to follow a plant-based diet for various health conditions

Here are some useful tips and advice on how to follow a plant-based diet for various health conditions:

1. If you have diabetes, you should try to eat more complex carbohydrates, such as whole grains, beans, fruits, and veggies, and less simple sugars, such as refined grains, sweets, and juices. You should also check your blood sugar levels regularly, and change your medicine, insulin, or diet as needed. You should also speak with your doctor or dietitian before making any changes to your food or medicine.

2. If you have heart disease, you should try to eat more unsaturated fats, such as nuts, seeds, avocados, and olive oil, and less saturated fats and trans fats, such as butter, cheese, cream, and fried foods. You should also limit your intake of salt, which can increase your blood pressure, and booze, which can increase your lipids. You should also check your blood pressure, cholesterol, and triglycerides regularly, and follow your doctor's advice on medicine, exercise, and diet.

3. If you have high blood pressure, you should try to eat more potassium-rich foods, such as bananas, potatoes, tomatoes, and beans, and less sodium-rich foods, such as processed foods, canned foods, and sauces. You should also limit your intake of caffeine, which can raise your blood pressure, and booze, which can interfere with your medicine. You should also check your blood pressure regularly, and follow your doctor's advice on medicine, exercise, and diet.

4. If you have high cholesterol, you should try to eat more soluble fiber, such as oats, apples, pears, and lentils, and less cholesterol-rich foods, such as eggs, meat, and cheese. You should also limit your intake of heavy fats and trans fats, which can increase your LDL cholesterol, and increase your intake of healthy fats and omega-3 fatty acids, which can increase your HDL cholesterol. You should also check your cholesterol numbers regularly, and follow your doctor's advice on medication, exercise, and diet.

These are some of the tips and information that I can give you on how to follow a plant-based diet for specific health problems. However, these are not meant to replace your doctor's or dietitian's suggestions, but rather to support them. You should always speak with your health care provider before making any changes to your diet or medicine, and follow their advice and supervision.

Success stories and testimonials

Success stories and comments from people who have better health with plant-based eating

To encourage and urge you to adopt a plant-based diet, I want to share with you some success stories and testimonials from people who have improved their health with plant-based eating. These are real people who have experienced real benefits from eating more plants and fewer animals. Here are some of their stories:

1. John, 56, from New York, fixed his type 2 diabetes and lost 60 pounds with a plant-based diet. He says: "I was diagnosed with type 2 diabetes in 2018, and I was prescribed metformin, insulin, and blood pressure medication. I was also overweight, unhappy, and tired all the time. I chose to try a plant-based diet after watching a program called Forks Over Knives, and I was amazed by the results. Within 3 months, I was able to stop taking all my medicines, and my blood sugar, blood pressure, and cholesterol were all normal. I also lost 60 pounds, got more energy, and felt happy and more confident. I never thought I could cure my

diabetes and change my life with a plant-based diet, but I did, and I'm never going back."

2. Mary, 62, from California, improved her cholesterol and blood pressure with a plant-based diet. She says: "I had high cholesterol and blood pressure for years, and I was taking statins and beta blockers to control them. I was also at risk of having a heart attack or a stroke, and I was scared for my health and my future. I chose to try a plant-based diet after reading a book called How Not to Die, and I was impressed by the science and the proof behind it. Within 6 months, I was able to drop my cholesterol by 100 points, and my blood pressure by 20 points, without any medicine. I also felt more energetic, lighter, and happy. I never thought I could lower my cholesterol and blood pressure with a plant-based diet, but I did, and I'm never going back."

3. David, 68, from Florida, helped his pain and asthma with a plant-based diet. He explains, "I've had arthritis and asthma for decades, and I used anti-inflammatory medicines and inhalers to treat them. I was also suffering from constant pain, stiffness, and shortness of breath, and I had trouble doing everyday tasks. I chose to try a plant-based diet after watching a video by Dr. Michael Greger, and I was intrigued by the benefits and the reviews. Within a year, I was able to lessen my

inflammation, pain, and medicine, and improve my mobility and breathing. I also felt more vibrant, young, and hopeful. I never thought I could improve my pain and asthma with a plant-based diet, but I did, and I'm never going back."

These are just some of the examples of the success stories and comments from people who have improved their health with plant-based eating. You can also be one of these success stories if you decide to give plant-based eating a try. You have nothing to lose, and everything to gain, by eating more plants and fewer animals.

Part 3: Plant-Based Eating for Enjoyment and Well-Being

Chapter 7: How to Make Plant-Based Eating Fun and Delicious

In this chapter, I'll show you how to make plant-based eating enjoyable and delectable, and how this can enhance your enjoyment and well-being. I'll also introduce some methods to add variety and flavor to your plant-based meals, teach some fundamental cooking skills and techniques that can enhance your plant-based dishes, and demonstrate some examples of how to make plant-based versions of your favorite foods.

How to add variety and flavor to your plant-based meals

One of the best ways to make plant-based dining enjoyable and delectable is to add variety and flavor to your plant-based meals. Variety and flavor can help you avoid boredom, satiate your taste receptors, and nourish your body and mind. Here are some methods to add variety and flavor to your plant-based meals:

Try new cuisines: Trying new cuisines can expose you to various flavors, ingredients, dishes, and cultures, that can enrich your plant-based dining experience. You can attempt cuisines that are inherently plant-based or plant-friendly, such as Asian, Indian, Mediterranean, or Mexican, or you can adapt cuisines that are traditionally animal-based, such as American, French, or Italian, to suit your plant-based preferences. You can experience new cuisines by visiting restaurants, ordering takeout, or cooking at home, using cookbooks, websites, or applications that can guide you through the recipes and techniques.

Try new ingredients: Trying new ingredients can introduce you to various textures, colors, shapes, and flavors, that can diversify your plant-based eating options. You can sample ingredients that are common or exotic, fresh or desiccated, whole or processed, depending on your availability and curiosity. You can try ingredients such as cereals, legumes, nuts, seeds, fruits, vegetables, herbs, seasonings, sauces, condiments, and more. You can sample new ingredients by perusing the grocery store, farmers market, or online store, or by joining a food delivery service, subscription box, or community-supported agriculture (CSA) program, that can deliver fresh and seasonal ingredients to your door.

Try new recipes: Trying new recipes can challenge you to create various dishes, meals, and menus that can vary your plant-based eating regimen. You can attempt recipes that are simple or complex, fast or sluggish, easy or hard, depending on your time and skill level. You can attempt recipes such as soups, salads, sandwiches, wraps, bowls, stir-fries, curries, casseroles, pies, cakes, pastries, and more.

fundamental cooking abilities and techniques that can enhance your plant-based dishes

One of the best ways to make plant-based dishes more delectable and satisfying is to acquire some fundamental cooking skills and techniques that can enhance their flavor, texture, and appearance. Here are some of the most common and useful cooking skills and techniques that you can apply to your plant-based dishes, along with some examples of how to use them.

Roasting: Roasting is a method of preparing food in an oven, using dry heat and high temperature. Roasting can help caramelize the natural sugars in food, creating a crusty, caramelized, and flavorful crust. Roasting can also help retain the moisture and tenderness of food, particularly vegetables, and tofu. Roasting is a straightforward and versatile technique that can be used for a variety of plant-based foods, such as potatoes, carrots, cauliflower, broccoli, Brussels sprouts, mushrooms, squash, eggplant, peppers, onions, garlic, tofu, tempeh, seitan, and more. To roast plant-based dishes, you will need a baking sheet, some oil or culinary spray, salt, pepper, and any other seasonings or herbs that you like. Preheat your oven to 375°F (190°C) and cut your food into bite-sized portions. Toss your food with oil or cooking spray, salt, pepper, and seasonings, and distribute them in an even layer on the baking sheet. Roast for 20 to 40 minutes, depending on the size and type of food, rotating halfway through, until caramelized and tender. Enjoy as a side dish, a main course, or a salad garnish.

Sautéing

Sautéing: Sautéing is a method of preparing food in a skillet, using a small quantity of oil or liquid and medium-high heat. Sautéing can help cook food swiftly and evenly, generating a seared, browned, and flavorful surface. Sautéing can also help unleash the aromas and flavors of food, particularly seasonings, herbs, and sauces. Sautéing is a rapid and simple technique that can be used for a variety of plant-based foods, such as onions, garlic, ginger, peppers, mushrooms, zucchini, spinach, kale, beans, lentils, chickpeas, tofu, tempeh, seitan, and more. To sauté plant-based dishes, you will need a skillet, some oil or bouillon, salt, pepper, and any other seasonings or sauces that you like. Heat your skillet over medium-high heat and add your oil or bouillon. Add your food and cook, stirring occasionally, for 10 to 15 minutes, depending on the size and type of food, until cooked through and caramelized. Season with salt, pepper, and any other seasonings or condiments that you like. Enjoy as a stir-fry, a curry, a fajita filling, or a sandwich stuffing.

Baking: Baking is a method of heating food in an oven, using dry heat and moderate temperature. Baking can help create a soft, moist, and fluffy texture in food, particularly breads, cakes, muffins, biscuits, and pies. Baking can also help create a golden, crusty, and flaky crust in food, particularly pastries, quiches, and pizzas. Baking is an enjoyable and inventive technique that can be used for a variety of plant-based foods, such as bananas, apples, berries, oats, almonds, seeds, flours, sugars, plant milk, plant yogurts, plant butter, plant cheeses, and more. To bake plant-based foods, you will need a baking dish, a mixing basin, a whisk, a spatula, some oil or cooking spray, and any other ingredients or utensils that your recipe requires. Preheat your oven to the temperature that your recipe specifies and lubricate your baking dish with oil or cooking spray. In a mixing basin, whisk together your liquid ingredients, such as plant milk, plant yogurt, plant butter, or flax eggs. In another basin, whisk together your dry ingredients, such as flour, sugar, baking powder, salt, and seasonings. Add your dry ingredients to your liquid ingredients and incorporate well with a spatula. Fold in any additional ingredients, such as fruits, almonds, seeds, or chocolate morsels. Transfer your mixture or dough to your baking dish and bake for the time that your recipe specifies until a toothpick inserted in the center comes out clean. Enjoy as a breakfast, a nibble, a dessert, or an indulgence.

examples of how to create plant-based variants of your beloved foods

One of the best ways to make plant-based eating enjoyable and delectable is to create plant-based versions of your beloved dishes, such as burgers, pizzas, pasta, desserts, and more. You can use plant-based ingredients to replace the animal products in your recipes, and still enjoy the same flavor, texture, and satisfaction. Here are some examples of how to make plant-based versions of your beloved foods:

Impossible Foods

Burgers: You can create plant-based burgers using legumes, lentils, chickpeas, tofu, tempeh, seitan, mushrooms, nuts, seeds, or grains, as the base. You can season them with seasonings, herbs, condiments, or vegan cheese, and shape them into patties. You can prepare them in a skillet, oven, or grill, and serve them on a bun, lettuce wrap, or salad, with your favorite garnishes, such as lettuce, tomato, onion, avocado, ketchup, mustard, or vegan mayo. You can also sample some of the plant-based burger brands that are available in the market, such as Beyond Meat, Impossible Foods, or Lightlife.

Pizzas: You can create plant-based pizzas using whole wheat, gluten-free, or cauliflower crusts, as the base. You can cover them with tomato sauce, pesto, hummus, or vegan cheese, and top them with your beloved vegetables, such as mushrooms, peppers, olives, artichokes, spinach, or broccoli. You can also add some plant-based proteins, such as tofu, tempeh, seitan, or vegan sausage, and sprinkle some vegan cheese, such as Daiya, Follow Your Heart, or Violife. You can bake them in the oven until the crust is golden and the cheese is softened, and savor them with some fresh basil, oregano, or red pepper flakes.

Pastas: You can create plant-based pastas using whole wheat, gluten-free, or bean-based noodles, as the substrate. You can mix them with your favorite sauces, such as marinara, alfredo, bolognese, or pesto, and add some vegetables, such as zucchini, eggplant, carrots, or peas. You can also add some plant-based proteins, such as legumes, lentils, chickpeas, tofu, tempeh, seitan, or vegan meatballs, and garnish with some vegan cheese, such as nutritional yeast, vegan parmesan, or vegan mozzarella. You can prepare them on the stovetop or in the oven, and savor them with some fresh parsley, basil, or thyme.

Desserts: You can create plant-based desserts using fruits, nuts, seeds, cereals, flours, sugars, plant milk, plant yogurts, plant butter, or plant cheeses, as the substrate. You can create cakes, pastries, muffins, pies, puddings, ice creams, or chocolates, using plant-based ingredients and sweeteners, such as maple syrup, agave nectar, or stevia. You can also add some flavors, such as vanilla, cinnamon, nutmeg, or cocoa, and some embellishments, such as chocolate morsels, nuts, seeds, or dried fruits. You can prepare them in the oven, chill them in the freezer, or blend them in the blender, and savor them with some whipped coconut cream, vegan caramel, or vegan frosting.

These are some of the examples of how to create plant-based versions of your beloved foods. You can find more recipes and ideas online or in books, magazines, or podcasts, that can help you create delectable and gratifying plant-based dishes. You can also experiment with your concoctions, using your creativity, intuition, and inspiration. You may be surprised by how simple and enjoyable it is to make plant-based versions of your beloved foods, and how good they taste and make you feel.

Chapter 8: How to Eat Plant-Based in Social Situations

In this chapter, I'll show you how to consume plant-based in social situations, and how this can enhance your enjoyment and well-being. I'll also acknowledge some of the challenges and opportunities of consuming plant-based food in social contexts, such as family gatherings, parties, restaurants, and more. I'll also propose some methods to communicate your dietary preferences and needs to others, offer some suggestions on how to prepare and plan ahead for social occasions, and encourage you to be flexible and appreciate the social aspect of eating, without compromising your health or values.

The challenges and opportunities of consuming plant-based in social settings

Eating plant-based in social contexts can be both challenging and rewarding, depending on the situation, the people, and your attitude. Some of the problems you may face include:

Lack of comprehension or support: You may encounter some people who do not understand or support your plant-based lifestyle, and who may question, disparage, or mock your choices. They may also attempt to persuade you to consume animal products or make you feel guilty or isolated for consuming differently.

Lack of options or availability: You may encounter some situations where plant-based options or availability are limited or nonexistent, such as family gatherings, parties, restaurants, or travel. You may also encounter some situations where plant-based options or availability are not explicitly labeled or communicated, such as buffets, potlucks, or menus.

Lack of convenience or comfort: You may encounter some situations where eating plant-based food is not convenient or comfortable, such as having to carry your own food, ask for special requests, or deny invitations. You may also encounter some situations where eating plant-based is not pleasurable or satisfying, such as having to consume bland or dull food, or losing out on your beloved foods.

Some of the opportunities that you may have are:

Sharing and learning: You may have the opportunity to share and learn about plant-based eating with others, such as explaining your reasons and benefits, providing data and resources, and recounting stories and experiences. You may also have the opportunity to learn from others, such as listening to their perspectives, opinions, and queries, and discovering new cuisines, ingredients, dishes, and flavors.

Finding and creating: You may have the opportunity to find and create plant-based options and availability in social contexts, such as researching and scouting for plant-based venues, ordering or preparing plant-based dishes, or suggesting or requesting plant-based alternatives. You may also have the opportunity to create your own plant-based options and availability, such as hosting or organizing plant-based events, inviting or joining plant-based groups, or initiating or supporting plant-based initiatives.

Enjoying and celebrating: You may have the opportunity to enjoy and celebrate plant-based eating in social contexts, such as sampling and relishing plant-based foods, expressing and appreciating gratitude, and having fun and creating memories. You may also have the opportunity to celebrate your plant-based dietary achievements, challenges, and changes, such as reaching your objectives, overcoming your barriers, and transforming your life.

How to communicate your dietary preferences and requirements to others

One of the most essential skills that you need to eat plant-based in social contexts is to communicate your dietary preferences and needs to others, in a manner that is polite, respectful, and confident. Here are some techniques to communicate your dietary preferences and requirements to others:

Be polite: Being polite means being courteous and considerate of others, and using appropriate words and etiquette. You can be courteous by stating please, thank you, and excuse me, and by using positive and friendly language. You can also be polite by avoiding interrupting, disputing, or complaining, and by respecting others' choices and opinions.

Be respectful: Being respectful means being mindful and appreciative of others, and acknowledging their emotions and perspectives. You can be respectful by listening and responding to others, and by demonstrating interest and empathy. You can also be respectful by avoiding judgment, criticizing, or shaming, and by accepting others' differences and diversity.

Be confident: Being confident means being assertive and self-assured of yourself, and expressing your needs and desires plainly and firmly. You can be confident by stating your plant-based preferences and requirements, and by explaining your reasons and benefits. You can also be confident by avoiding apologizing, justifying, or concealing, and by standing up for yourself and your values.

How to prepare and plan ahead for social occasions

One of the most useful tips that you can use to consume plant-based in social contexts is to prepare and plan ahead for social occasions, in a way that is practical, flexible, and creative. <u>Here are some tips on how to prepare and plan ahead for social occasions:</u>

Bring your own food: taking your own food means preparing and packaging your own plant-based food, and taking it with you to social occasions. You can bring your own food by creating or purchasing plant-based dishes, munchies, or desserts, and preserving them in containers, bags, or coolers. You can also bring your own food by offering or volunteering to bring plant-based cuisine to share with others, such as for potlucks, picnics, or parties.

Check menus: Checking menus means researching and perusing the menus of the restaurants or venues that you are going to visit, and looking for plant-based options or availability. You can check menus by visiting the websites, calling the phone numbers, or asking the staff of the restaurants or venues, and find out what plant-based dishes, ingredients, or alternatives they offer. You can also check menus by using applications, websites, or guides that can help you discover plant-based restaurants or venues, such as HappyCow, VeggieBoards, or VegGuide.

Ask questions: Asking questions means inquiring and requesting information or clarification about the plant-based options or availability of the food that you are going to consume, and making sure that they meet your preferences and requirements. You can ask inquiries by chatting to the hostesses, visitors, servers, or chefs of the social occasions, and finding out what the food contains, how it is produced, or if it can be modified. You can also ask inquiries by using considerate and respectful language, such as "Do you have any plant-based options?" "What are the ingredients of this dish?" or "Can you please make this dish without cheese?"

Be flexible and appreciate the social aspect of eating
One of the most important strategies that you can use to consume plant-based in social contexts is to be flexible and appreciate the social aspect of dining, without compromising your health or values. Being flexible and appreciating the social aspect of eating means being open-minded and adaptable to various situations and people and focusing on the positive and enjoyable aspects of dining with others, rather than the negative and stressful ones. **Here are some methods to be flexible and appreciate the social aspect of eating:**

Be flexible: Being flexible means being willing and able to alter your expectations and preferences, and to make the best of what is available and possible. You can be flexible by acknowledging that not every social occasion will be optimal or ideal for your plant-based eating, and by being prepared to deal with some challenges or inconveniences. You can also be flexible by being creative and resourceful, and by discovering or creating plant-based options or alternatives, even if they are not obvious or simple. You can also be flexible by being grateful and appreciative, and by acknowledging and savoring what you have, rather than what you don't have.

Enjoy the social aspect of eating: Enjoying the social aspect of eating means being mindful and attentive to the people and the atmosphere and to the delight and joy of dining with others, rather than to the food and the diet. You can appreciate the social aspect of dining by engaging and connecting with others, and by sharing and learning about plant-based eating, or other topics of interest. You can also appreciate the social aspect of dining by having fun and celebrating, and by creating and cherishing memories, rather than by worrying or stressing about your food choices. You can also appreciate the social aspect of eating by being proud and confident, and by expressing and honoring your health and values, rather than by concealing or compromising them.

By being flexible and appreciating the social aspect of dining, you can make plant-based eating in social settings more enjoyable and delicious, and less challenging and stressful.

You can also enhance your enjoyment and well-being, and inspire and influence others, by consuming more flora and fewer animals.

Chapter 9: How to Cultivate a Positive Relationship with Food and Yourself

In this chapter, I'll show you how to develop a positive relationship with food and yourself, and how this can improve your enjoyment and well-being. I'll also talk about the importance of having a healthy and balanced attitude towards food and eating, especially as you age. I'll also address some common problems and worries that older people may face, such as body image, weight, appetite, and more. I'll also provide some tactics and practices to cope with these problems and concerns, such as mindfulness, gratitude, self-compassion, and more. I'll also tell you that eating plant-based is not only good for your physical health, but also for your mental and social well-being.

The importance of having a healthy and balanced approach to food and eating

Food is more than just power for your body. Food is also a source of happiness, comfort, culture, and relationship. Food can feed your body, mind, and soul, and help you live a longer, happy, and healthier life. However, food can also become a source of worry, guilt, shame, and strife, if you have an unhealthy and unbalanced approach towards food and eating. A bad and unbalanced approach towards food and eating can affect your health, feelings, and quality of life, especially as you age. Some signs of a harmful and unbalanced approach towards food and eating are:

1. Obsessing over calories, nutrients, or amounts
2. Restricting or avoiding certain foods or food groups
3. Binging or overeating on certain foods or food groups
4. Feeling bad or worried after eating
5. Comparing your body or eating habits to others
6. Judging yourself or others based on food choices or body size
7. Using food to cope with anxiety, boredom, loneliness, or other feelings
8. Ignoring your hunger, fullness, or pleasure cues
9. Neglecting your health, cleanliness, or social needs because of food

<u>Having a good and balanced approach towards food and eating means that you can:</u>

1. Enjoy a range of foods that provide you with the nutrients and energy you need
2. Listen to your body and eat according to your hunger, fullness, and pleasure cues
3. Respect your food tastes and wants, and respect your cravings and appetites
4. Appreciate the taste, texture, scent, and look of food

5. Celebrate the cultural, social, and emotional sides of food

6. Accept your body and eating habits, and respect your skills and abilities

7. Be flexible and adjustable to different events and people

8. Be aware and attentive to your food and eating situations

9. Be grateful and caring to yourself and others

<u>Having a good and balanced approach towards food and eating can help you:</u>

1. Prevent or control chronic diseases, such as diabetes, heart disease, high blood pressure, high cholesterol, and more

2. Maintain or improve your physical ability, movement, and balance

3. Support your immunity system, nutrition, and metabolism

4. Enhance your happiness, memory, and reasoning

5. Reduce your worry, anxiety, and sadness

6. Increase your self-esteem, confidence, and happiness

7. Strengthen your connections, communication, and social skills

8. Improve your quality of life and well-being

The common problems and worries that older adults may face

As you age, you may face some problems and worries that can affect your food and eating habits, such as:

Physical factors: Aging can cause changes in your body that can affect your hunger, digestion, metabolism, and nutrition needs. For example, you may experience a decrease in your sense of taste, smell, or thirst, which can make food less appealing or fulfilling. You may also have dental problems, swallowing issues, or chronic diseases, which can make eating more challenging or painful. You may also need to change your diet or medication, based on your health state or doctor's advice.

Social factors: Aging can also cause changes in your social surroundings that can affect your food and eating habits. For example, you may experience a lack of social contact, such as retirement, the death of a spouse or friend, or relocation, which can make you feel lonely or solitary. You may also have less access to food, transportation, or cooking tools, which can limit your food choices or availability. You may also face social pressure, stigma, or abuse, based on your food decisions or body size.

Emotional factors: Aging can also cause changes in your emotional state that can affect your food and eating habits. For example, you may feel sadness, anxiety, grief, or boredom, which can affect your mood, motivation, or interest in food. You may also use food to deal with your moods, which can lead to emotional eating, binge eating, or overeating. You may also have bad thoughts or views about yourself, your body, or your food, which can affect your self-esteem, confidence, or happiness.

These problems and concerns can make it hard for you to have a good and balanced approach towards food and eating and can affect your health, emotions, and quality of life. However, you can beat these challenges and cope with these issues and concerns, by using some tactics and practices that can help you.

The strategies and techniques to cope with these problems and worries

There are many techniques and practices that can help you deal with the problems and concerns that you may face as you age, and help you have a healthy and balanced approach towards food and eating. Here are some of them:

Seek professional help: If you have a medical, nutritional, or mental health issue that affects your food and eating habits, such as diabetes, heart disease, depression, or an eating disorder, you should seek professional help from a doctor, dietitian, therapist, or other qualified healthcare provider. They can help you diagnose, treat, and manage your condition, and provide you with the proper advice, support, and tools that you need.

Seek social support: If you feel lonely, separated, or ignored, you should seek social support from your family, friends, neighbors, or community. They can help you feel connected, respected, and cared for, and provide you with the mental, practical, and financial assistance that you need. You can also join social groups, clubs, or events that interest you, and meet new people who share your skills, passions, or goals.

Seek information and education: If you feel confused, unsure, or misled about food and eating, you should seek information and education from trusted sources, such as books, websites, or podcasts, that can help you learn more about nutrition, health, and well-being. You can also attend programs, classes, or courses that can teach you new skills, such as cooking, gardening, or meditation, that can improve your food and eating experiences.

Practice mindfulness: Mindfulness is the practice of paying attention to the current moment, with curiosity, openness, and acceptance. You can practice awareness by focusing on your breath, body, sensations, thoughts, feelings, or surroundings, and watching them without judgment or response. You can also practice mindful eating, which is the practice of eating with focus, purpose, and attention. You can practice mindful eating by eating slowly, chewing well, savoring the flavors, noticing the textures, and listening to your hunger, fullness, and pleasure signs.

Practice gratitude: Gratitude is the practice of showing thankfulness for what you have, rather than what you don't have. You can practice thankfulness by writing down or saying out loud what you are grateful for, such as your food, your body, your health, your family, your friends, or your life. You can also practice gratitude by showing kindness, generosity, or care to yourself and others, such as by giving praise, gifts, or help, or by saying thank you, sorry, or I love you.

Practice self-compassion: Self-compassion is the practice of treating yourself with kindness, understanding, and acceptance, rather than with criticism, blame, or shame. You can practice self-compassion by recognizing your feelings, needs, and struggles, and by giving yourself approval, comfort, and care. You can also practice self-compassion by speaking to yourself in a gentle, helpful, and encouraging way, rather than in a harsh, negative, or depressing way.

These tactics and practices can help you deal with the problems and concerns that you may face as you age, and help you have a healthy and balanced approach towards food and eating. They can also help you improve your health, feelings, and quality of life, and help you enjoy food and eating more.

The benefits of eating plant-based for your mental and emotional well-being

Eating plant-based is not only good for your physical health, but also for your mental and social well-being. Eating plant-based can help you:

Boost your mood: Eating plant-based can help you boost your mood, as plant foods are rich in vitamins, phytochemicals, and omega-3 fatty acids, which can help reduce inflammation, oxidative stress, and sadness. Plant foods are also high in fiber, complex carbohydrates, and tryptophan, which can help balance your blood sugar, insulin, and serotonin levels, and help you feel more calm, happy, and pleased.

Enhance your cognition: Eating plant-based can help you enhance your cognition, as plant foods are rich in vitamins, minerals, and phytochemicals, that can help protect your brain cells, synapses, and neurons, and help you improve your memory, learning, and focus. Plant foods are also low in saturated fat, cholesterol, and trans fat, which can help avoid or slow cognitive decline, dementia, and Alzheimer's disease.

Increase your self-esteem: Eating plant-based can help you increase your self-esteem, as plant foods are low in calories, fat, and sodium, and high in fiber, water, and nutrients, which can help you maintain or achieve a healthy weight, lower your blood pressure, and improve your skin, hair, and nails. Plant foods are also ethical.

Conclusion

Congratulations! You have finished the 30-day plant-based challenge and learned how to eat plant-based for health, life, and happiness. You have also found how to make plant-based eating fun, delicious, and satisfying, and how to deal with the difficulties and opportunities of eating plant-based in social settings. You have also developed a good relationship with food and yourself and experienced the benefits of eating plant-based food for your physical, mental, and emotional well-being.

<u>Here are some of the important points and lessons from this book:</u>

- Eating plant-based means eating more foods that are derived from plants, such as fruits, veggies, grains, beans, nuts, and seeds, and eating less or no foods that are derived from animals, such as meat, dairy, eggs, and fish.
1. Eating plant-based can help you avoid or manage chronic diseases, such as diabetes, heart disease, high blood pressure, high cholesterol, and more, by providing you with the nutrients, antioxidants,

phytochemicals, and fiber that your body needs to work properly and ideally.

2. Eating plant-based food can also help you support your healthy aging, by improving your immune system, digestion, metabolism, brain, and physical function, and by lowering your inflammation, oxidative stress, and risk of cognitive decline, dementia, and Alzheimer's disease.

3. Eating plant-based can also help you improve your mood, memory, and happiness, by regulating your blood sugar, insulin, and serotonin levels, and by giving you omega-3 fatty acids, tryptophan, and vitamin B12, which can help lower depression, anxiety, and stress.

4. Eating plant-based can also help you boost your self-esteem, confidence, and happiness, by helping you keep or achieve a healthy weight, lower your blood pressure, improve your skin, hair, and nails, and by aligning your food choices with your values, ethics, and beliefs.

5. Eating plant-based can also help you enjoy and celebrate food and eating, by presenting you with new cuisines, ingredients, dishes, and flavors, by teaching you new skills, techniques, and recipes, and by connecting you with other people, cultures, and feelings.

You have done a great job of eating plant-based for 30 days, and I hope you are proud of yourself and your accomplishments. You have also taken a big step towards improving your health, happiness, and well-being, and I hope you are feeling the good results of eating plant-based. You have also started a trip that can last a lifetime, and I hope you are excited to continue it.

Eating plant-based is not a diet, but a lifestyle. It is not a limit, but a choice. It is not a loss, but a joy. Eating plant-based is not only good for you, but also for the animals, the earth, and the world. Eating plant-based is a way of life that can help you live longer, happy, and healthier.

I hope this book has inspired and pushed you to eat plant-based, and to enjoy the benefits and joys of eating more plants and fewer animals. I hope this book has also given you the information, advice, and support that you need to eat plant-based successfully and sustainably. I hope this book has also helped you to have a healthy and balanced attitude towards food and eating, and to develop a good relationship with food and yourself.

Thank you for reading this book, and thank you for taking the 30-day plant-based challenge. You have made a change in your life and in the lives of others.

www.ingramcontent.com/pod-product-compliance
Lightning Source LLC
Chambersburg PA
CBHW070819260726
48660CB00005B/1905